The Revolutionary Keto Diet

The Ultimate Cookbook for Weight Loss and a Healthy Lifestyle

By

Angel Burns

License Notices

Table of Contents

Introduction

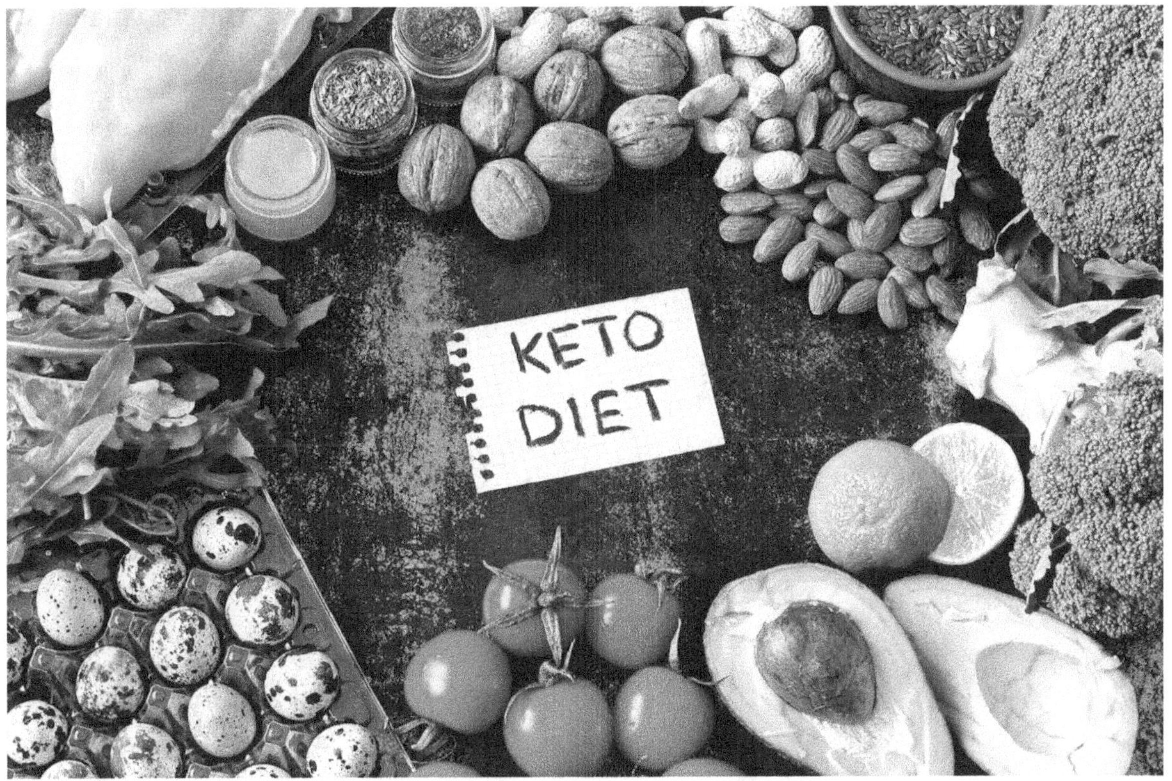

Starting a new diet is a process that comes with a lot of questions, no matter what the diet is or who is starting it. Making severe changes to one's diet can be stressful and confusing, but it doesn't have to be. If a person does adequate research on their desired diet before jumping in head first, they can start the program feeling intelligent, competent, and confident.

Keto can seem like one of those diets that is difficult to wrap one's head around, and even some people who are on a diet don't fully understand the mechanics and benefits surrounding it. Although it is a fairly straightforward diet, once a person is accustomed to it, it can be confusing for beginners to determine how to get the correct amount of nutrients and which foods contain the nutrients they need. This guide teaches aspiring Keto dieters the ins and outs of the diet so they can put their fears behind them and embark on possibly the best decision they can make for their health.

The Ketogenic Diet

Keto diet is a low carbohydrate that has a high percentage of fat in the diet that enables the body to produce ketoses in the liver and make use of them as energy. More so, the main source of generating energy for our body is glucose because when you consume something that is high in carbohydrates the body system will process them into glucose.

By eating fewer carbs, you induce your body to the state of ketosis thus making it easier for the body to tap into the stored fat reserves it already has on hand. But getting yourself into the state of ketosis is never easy. Either you go on fasting for days or you cut down your carb intake to 50 grams daily, which is equivalent to around 5% of your total calories.

This can be achieved by changing your diet. Instead of taking in your usual diet, you can drive ketosis by eating more fat and protein. Your fat should be 60-75% of your daily calories while your protein intake should be 15-30% of your calories. This is equivalent to 1 large chicken breast and 5 small avocados each meal. Because fat is naturally filling, it will keep you full for a long time, so you will not feel the need to snack between meals.

The goal for the Ketogenic diet is to get your body into the state of ketosis by breaking down fats into ketones as the primary source of fuel by eating the right amounts of food that support such metabolic pathways.

Low carbs are only one aspect of the Keto Diet. It not only leads you on your way to losing weight, but it also takes your body to an enhanced state of health and well-being. You feel stronger and more energized, which means no unhealthy snacks can sneak up on you when you have hunger pangs. You control your eating, but you are eating better and healthier.

It's for these reasons that so many people around the world are embracing this amazing diet. Its scientific underpinnings ensure that it works. Ketogenic is not a term coined by some new-age guru, it is a scientifically proven process with nearly a hundred years of history that has been validated and tested by many studies and researches.

Ketosis is a state when, in the absence of carbohydrates, your body is compelled to use the alternative source of energy and it burns the fats stored in your body for this purpose. That is why the Keto Diet has been so successful. This is not something new, it has been around for ages.

The ancient Indian physicians used to fast for days, which led to ketosis which they saw enriched their minds and bodies. Since the early 1920s, the Keto Diet was used to treat and help epileptic children.

The Keto Diet is a process which, like any other process, is difficult in the beginning because you are trying to break habits that have been formed over the years. But once you go through the process, you see a healthier and stronger you. Another feature that makes Keto stand out is that there is no deprivation or hunger involved. You do not stop eating; you choose to eat in a better and healthier way.

Benefits of Keto

Keto diet comes with many health benefits, even though many people attempt the diet for the sole purpose of weight loss. It has the capacity to bring about beneficial changes to the human body. Many of the health benefits users can expect with the Keto diet are:

Weight loss

This is the reason for the widespread acceptance of the Keto diet. When you start with the Keto diet, the body loses many of its water which translates to fat loss due to decreased intake of carb.

When carb intake goes down as well, the blood sugar level goes down. As a result, the body enjoys steady energy levels. This also translates to a reduction in hunger, removing the need to snack now and then. The ability to keep users full helps in reducing craving and desire to eat.

This scarcity of glucose through a reduction in carb intake causes the body to burn more fat for energy.

You are in Control of Your Appetite

In time as you proceed with the Keto diet, your rate of hunger and cravings subside considerably. As a result, many Keto dieters find intermittent fasting pretty easy. This is due to the reduction in the rate of hunger. Even with limited food intake, your energy level is still intact since your body is powered by fat.

Improved Mental Focus

This is one of the many positive changes users experience in starting the Keto diet. Some source of healthy fats contains omega 3 fatty acids like tuna, mackerel, and salmon. These rewards users with improved mood and high learning capacity. The brain contains a fair percentage of DHA (15 to 30%). Consuming omega-3 fatty acids makes this fatty acid increase, rewarding the brain.

Beta-hydroxybutyrate is a type of ketone produced during ketosis which helps improve memory function.

Also, one of the disadvantages of using carb is that it causes the rise and fall in the blood sugar levels. This causes inconsistency in the energy level, which makes it difficult for the brain to focus. With a consistent energy source like ketone, the brain can focus.

Insulin Sensitivity

When the insulin level in the body is too high, it causes insulin resistance. Keto diet can help with this as meals high in carb generally trigger high insulin resistance.

With a low carb diet, on the other hand, insulin level falls. We can attribute this to the increase in the level of fat, a macronutrient that doesn't thrive with insulin.

When the insulin level goes down, the body can burn more fat because excess insulin restricts the breakdown of fats.

Better Control of Blood Pressure

Many people, in our world today are dealing with increased blood pressure. This results in several other health issues like stroke, kidney failure, and heart disease.

The Keto diet, however, comes as a savior to reduce high blood pressure. This is why the Keto diet works wonder for people with type 2 diabetes or people with obesity.

Increased Energy Level

The body is not evolved to store glycogen. This means that the body needs to keep stocking the level up to help maintain the energy level.

Adopting the Keto diet changes this as the body now depends on fat, which is available in excess. As a result, you will hardly run out of fuel when you are in ketosis.

Helps Control Epilepsy

The discovery of a Keto diet is tied to the control of epilepsy. Centuries ago, the main focus of the Keto diet was in treating victims of epilepsy. Victims experienced a significant decrease in the rate of seizures when placed on the diet.

Can Help You get to Autophagy

If you want to live long, grow old without being subjected to health issues that come with old age, the Keto diet can help you. This is because getting to ketosis is one of the most effective ways to trigger autophagy. The other two are intermittent fasting and intense exercise. With autophagy, the body gets the ability to either expel or recycle worn out and damaged body cells. This leads to the growth of new and strong cells, rewarding you with a vibrant and healthy body, which can fight diseases and pathogens.

Foods to Avoid.

The Ketogenic diet is not rocket science. While it limits what type of foods that you can consume, it is not really difficult to eliminate certain food groups from your meals. This diet is a very restrictive one that does not allow eating certain foods such as grains, rice, beans, potatoes, sweets, cereals and some fruits. Avoid the following

Grains or starches: Grains and starches are broken down into glucose thus they should be avoided at all costs. These include rice, pasta, oatmeal, rye, barley, wheat-based products, cereal, corn, and basically all types of grains imaginable.

Beans/legumes: Peas, chickpeas, lentils, etc. Beans and legumes are high in starch thus it is converted into glucose.

Root vegetables and tubers: Carrots, sweet potatoes, parsnips, etc. They contain high amounts of starch, which can be converted into simple sugar.

Fruit: All fruits with exception of some berries like strawberries. Fruits contain high amounts of fructose.

Sugary foods: Candy, soda, cakes, etc.

Sugar of all types: These include honey, maple syrup, white sugar, brown sugar, molasses, and fruit sugars.

Unhealthy fats/Processed oils: Limit your intake of processed vegetable oils, mayonnaise, etc. Ketogenic diet advocates the consumption of healthy fats, but it discourages the consumption of processed oils such as vegetable oil, canola oil, corn oil, and soy oil.

Soda and fruit juice: Soda and fruit juice (yes, even the natural kind) are full of sugar such as glucose and fructose so they can kick you out of ketosis.

Snacks: Your favorite snacks such as donuts, cookies, cakes, and chocolate bars are strictly prohibited when you are following the Ketogenic diet as they are loaded with a lot of sugar and trans-fat.

Alcohol.

Foods to Eat

Staying in ketosis by eating the right foods is key to healthy weight loss. It is important that you consume more healthy fats than protein to stay in this particular metabolic pathway. I will constantly stress the importance of following the percentage of 5% carbs, 20% protein, and 75% fats. This means that you need to build your meals around low carb vegetables, healthy oils, and moderate protein. Below are the foods that you can consume to drive ketosis.

Fatty fish: Fatty fish is a great source of fatty acids like Omega-3s that are precursors to ketones. Source them from trout, sardines, salmon, tuna, mackerel, herring, and mostly cold-water fishes as they have more Omega-3s than other fishes.

Meat: Choose from a selection of red meats, pork or ham, steak, sausage, bacon, chicken, turkey, and organ meats. Consume only a matchbox-sized portion for this diet regimen.

Grass fed Butter and cream.

Pastured Eggs.

Unprocessed cheese like cheddar or mozzarella.

Healthy oils like olive oil (extra virgin), avocado oil.

Nuts and seeds: Nuts and seeds are stapled food items among Keto dieters. Almonds, walnuts, flax seeds, cashew nuts, brazil nuts, pumpkin seeds, chia seeds, etc.

Avocados: Whole avocados or freshly made guacamole.

Low-carb veggies/Vegetables growing above ground: Low carb vegetables in the form of leafy greens, cucumbers, onions, tomatoes, broccoli, cauliflower, and peppers are allowed in this diet. Basically, all vegetables growing above ground (except some squash varieties and tomatoes) are mostly made up of fiber, water, and less sugar.

Good fats: Remember that not all fats are created equally. While some fats are bad, some are very healthy for the body. You need to consume more good fats in the Ketogenic diet. Your options include MCT oil, coconut oil, butter, olive oil, ghee, avocado oil, and other dairy sources like unprocessed cheese, and cream. Another good source of healthy fat is avocado.

Berries: While most fruits are high discouraged while following the Ketogenic diet, there are low sugar fruits that you are allowed to eat, and these include blueberries, limes, lemons, apples, and strawberries.

Sweeteners: Sweeteners sourced from sugar with a high glycemic index is bad for the Ketogenic diet. However, allowed sweeteners include stevia, monk fruits, and erythritol.

Water: Water is the most acceptable beverage in the Ketogenic diet because it contains no calories. But if you are not such a big fan of this particular diet, you can always opt for other beverages such as tea, coffee, and red wine (occasionally).

Bone broth: Bone broth is not only hydrating but it is also chockfull of electrolytes, healthy fats, and nutrients. It is a great beverage to sip on the Keto diet. For added fat, add a small dollop of butter to jump start ketosis.

Breakfast Recipes

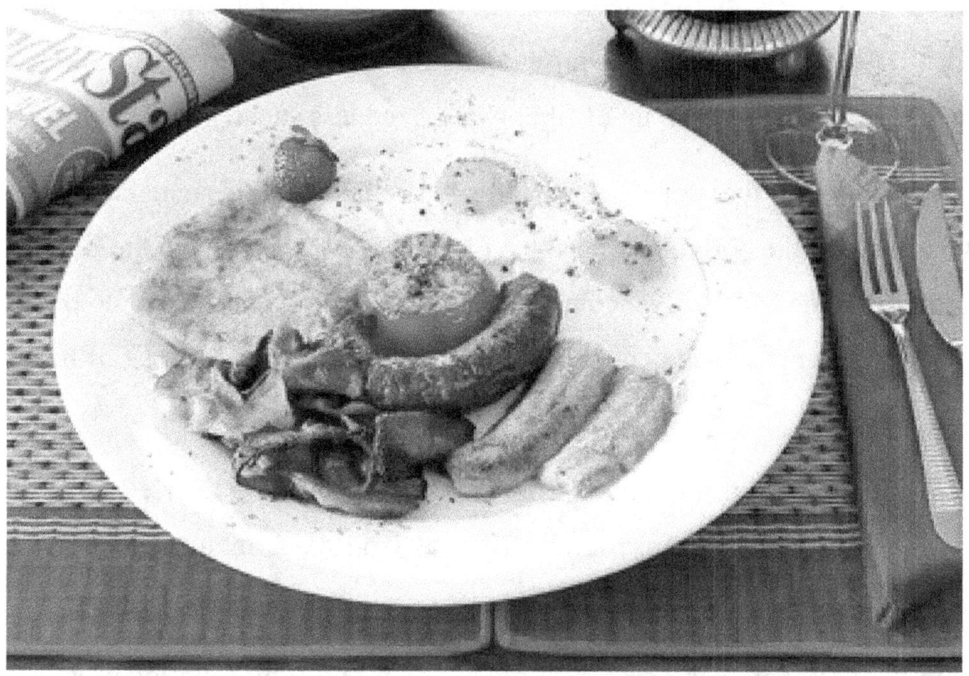

Breakfast is an important part of having your meals on a daily basis. To start off your day in style, all you need is to strategize on a number of meals that will keep you energized and strengthened all through. This diet has a wonderful collection of recipes that will ensure proper health for everyone, inclusive of non-family members. Let everyone enjoy the sweetness and health that comes from this specially chosen Keto diet breakfast recipes.

Chocolate and Peanut Butter Smoothie

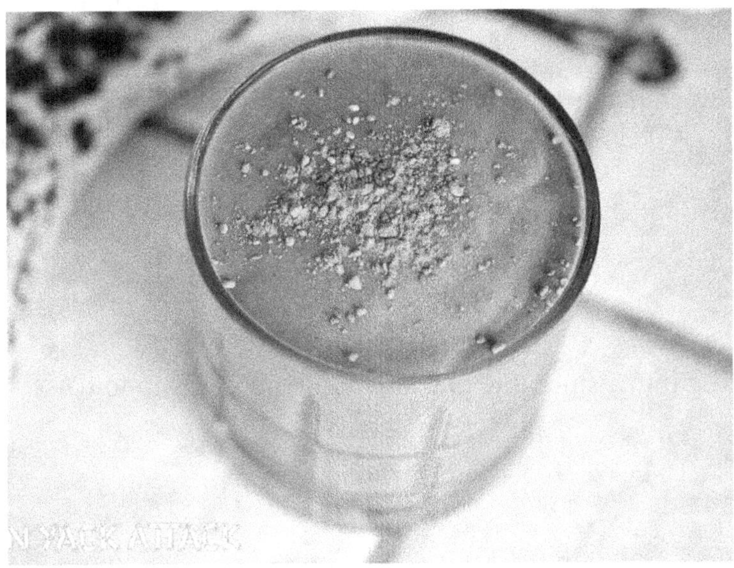

You will always love starting your morning in style with the Chocolate and Peanut Butter Smoothie. The smoothie provides a great way of commencing your day in an energized manner. Enjoy it!

Servings: 1

Cooking time: 5 mins

Ingredients:

- 1 c. coconut milk, unsweetened
- 1tbsp. cocoa powder, unsweetened
- 1tbsp. unsweetened peanut butter
- 5 drops stevia
- 1 pinch salt

Instructions:

1. Chuck everything into a smoothie maker, and blend until smooth.

2. Serve immediately.

Cream Cheese and Cinnamon Pancakes

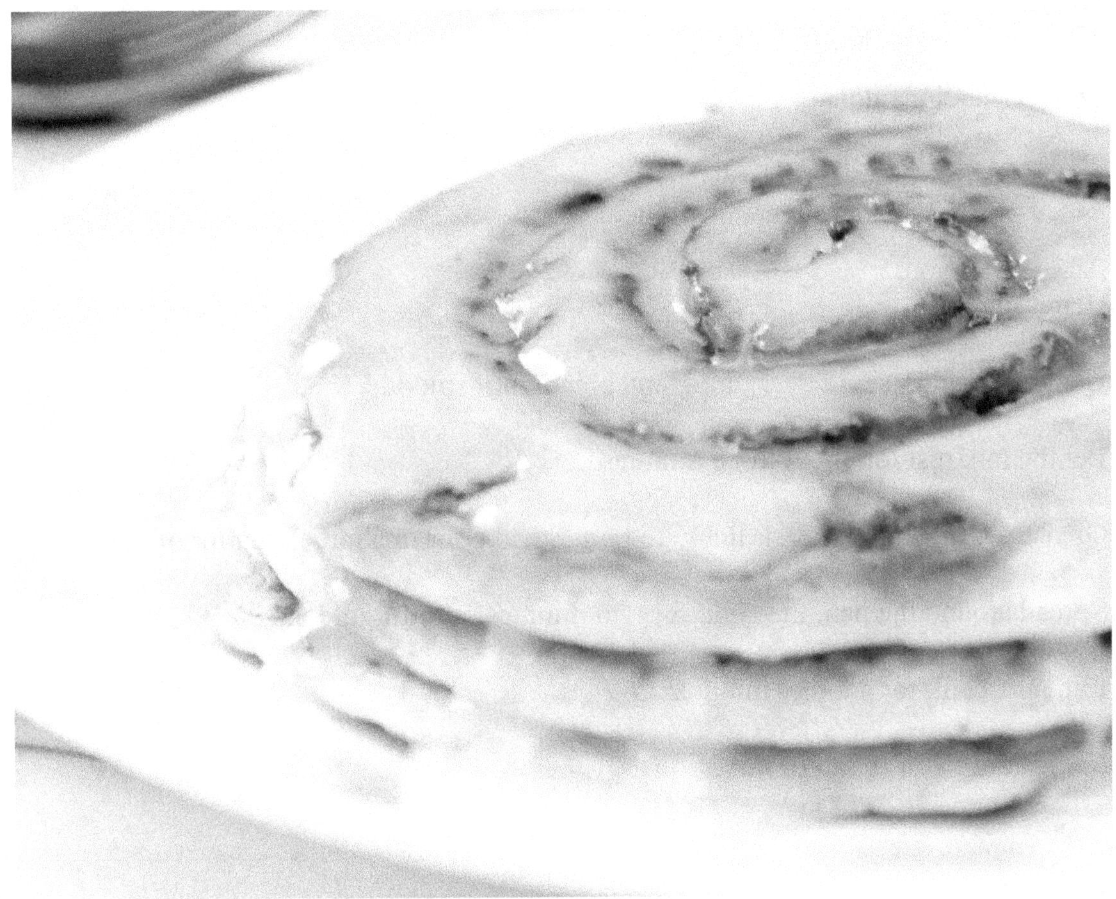

For a delicious homemade pancake, a try of Cream Cheese and Cinnamon cakes can be quite amazing. It is purely deliciousness.

Servings: 4

Cooking time: 12 mins

Ingredients:

- 2 eggs
- 2 oz. cream cheese
- ½ tsp. cinnamon
- ½ c. almond flour
- 1 tsp. granulated sugar substitute

Instructions:

1. Using a blender, set in everything and blend until smooth.

2. Let the mix rest for about three minutes.

3. Grease a large, non-stick skillet with butter, and pour in about a quarter of the mix.

4. Spread around the pan, the cook for two minutes or until golden.

5. Flip, and cook for another minute.

6. Repeat until you're out of mix.

Chia and Honey Coconut Pudding

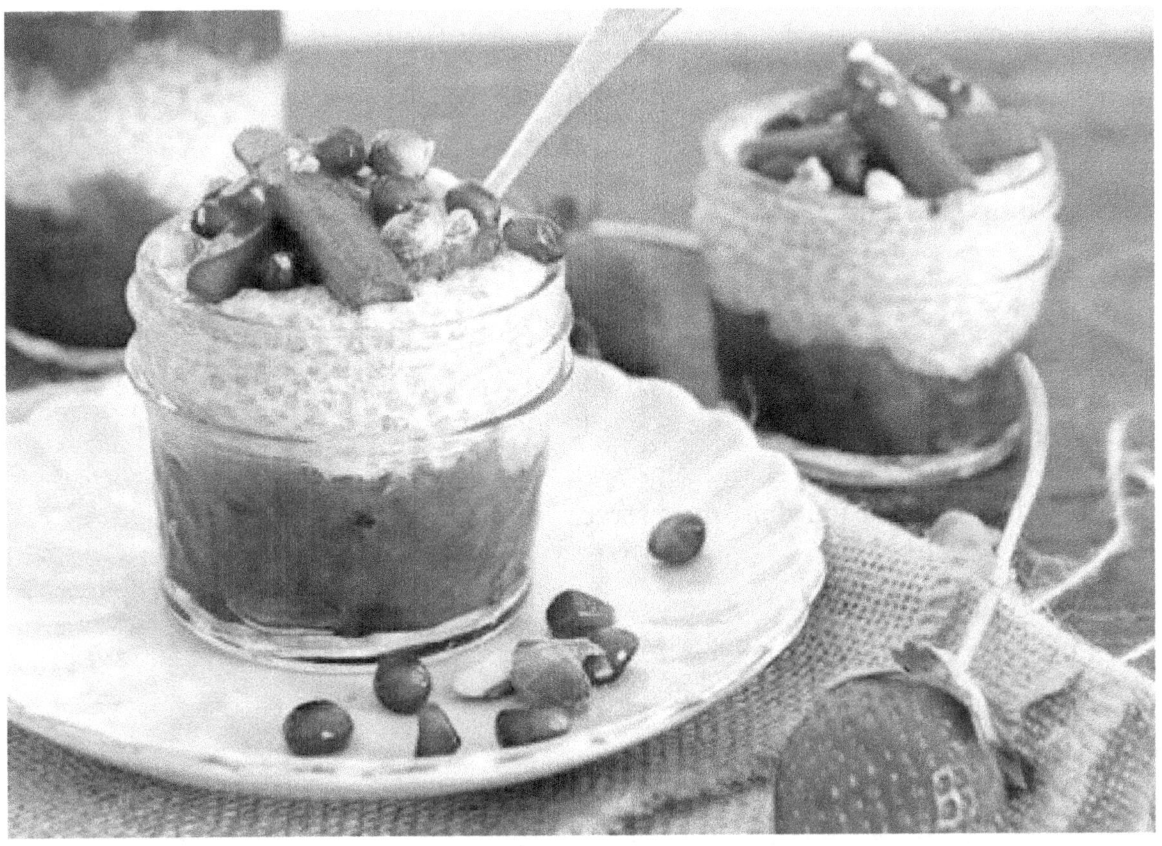

The pudding is a good one health-wise and is loaded with lots of essential ingredients to ensure your health is not at stake. Enjoy!

Servings: 4

Cooking time: 25 mins

Ingredients:

- ½ tbsp. honey
- 1 c. full-fat coconut milk
- ¼ c. chia seeds
- ¼ c. raspberries
- 2 tbsps. almonds

Instructions:

1. In a bowl, stir together the honey, chia seeds, and coconut milk. Leave to chill overnight in the fridge.

2. Top with raspberries and almonds to serve.

Turkey and Cauliflower Hash

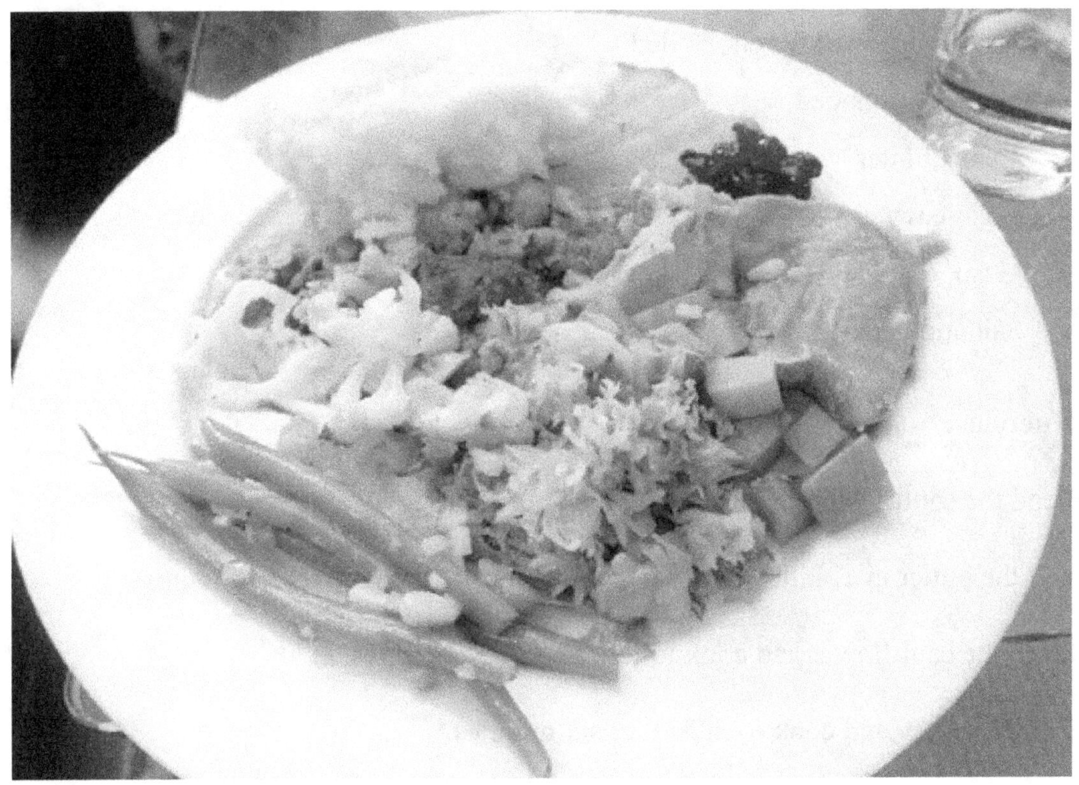

Try and make yourself a healthy and perfect treat by preparing the Turkey and Cauliflower Hash meal. It is simple and easy and hence no need to strain while preparing it.

Servings: 2

Cooking time: 30 mins

Ingredients:

- ½ lb. cooked turkey, chopped
- ½ c. cauliflower florets, boiled
- ½ onion, chopped
- 1 tbsp. butter
- ¼ c. heavy cream
- ½ tsp. dried and crushed thyme
- Salt and pepper

Instructions:

1. Blend the cauliflower until crumbly, then put aside.

2. Melt the butter in a skillet, then sauté the onions for around three minutes.

3. Stir in the cauliflower and cook for another three minutes.

4. Add the turkey and cook for a further six minutes.

5. Stir in the heavy cream and cook for another 2 minutes, stirring constantly.

6. Serve immediately or keep in the fridge for up to three days.

Scrambled Eggs with Tomatoes and Chili Pepper

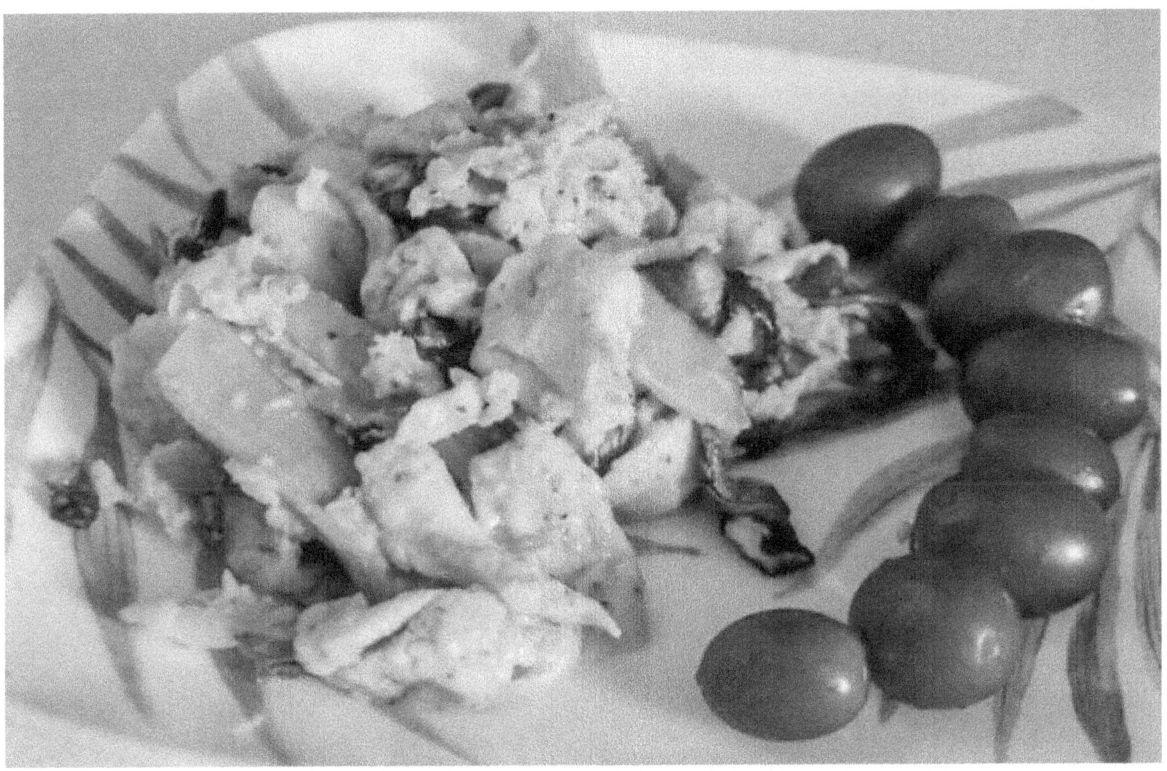

A dish that majorly entails a mixture of scrambled eggs, tomatoes, chili pepper, and other ingredients is quite amazing. Enjoy it.

Servings: 2

Cooking time: 20 mins

Ingredients:

- 4 organic eggs
- 2 tbsps. scallions, sliced thinly
- 1 chopped tomato
- 1 Serrano chili pepper
- 2 tbsps. cilantro, chopped finely
- ¼ c. heavy cream
- 3 tbsps. butter
- Salt and pepper

Instructions:

1. In a bowl, beat the eggs with the cilantro and salt and pepper.

2. In a pan over a medium heat, melt the butter and cook the tomatoes and chili pepper for around two minutes.

3. Pour in the egg, and cook for four minutes, stirring continuously.

4. Serve topped with fresh scallions.

Cheesy Cauliflower Waffles

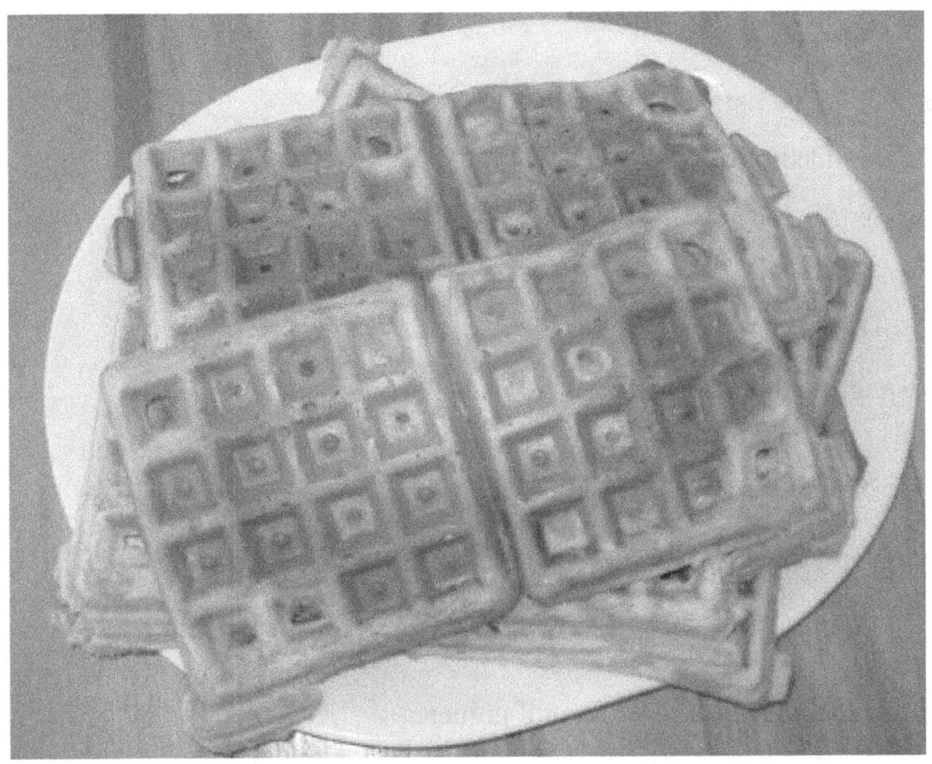

Enrich yourself with a morning packed with cheesy cauliflower waffles. The waffles are healthy and will energize you as you start your day.

Servings: 2

Cooking time: 20 mins

Ingredients:

- 2 eggs, beaten
- 1 c. cauliflower
- ½ c. shredded parmesan cheese
- 1 c. shredded mozzarella cheese
- 1 tsp. garlic powder
- 1 tsp. onion powder
- 1 tbsp. minced chives
- ½ tsp. ground black pepper

Instructions:

1. Mix everything together in a bowl.

2. Prep your waffle iron by greasing and pre-heating it.

3. Pour in half the mixture and cook until golden.

4. Repeat with the remaining mixture.

5. Serve.

Spinach and Bacon Frittata

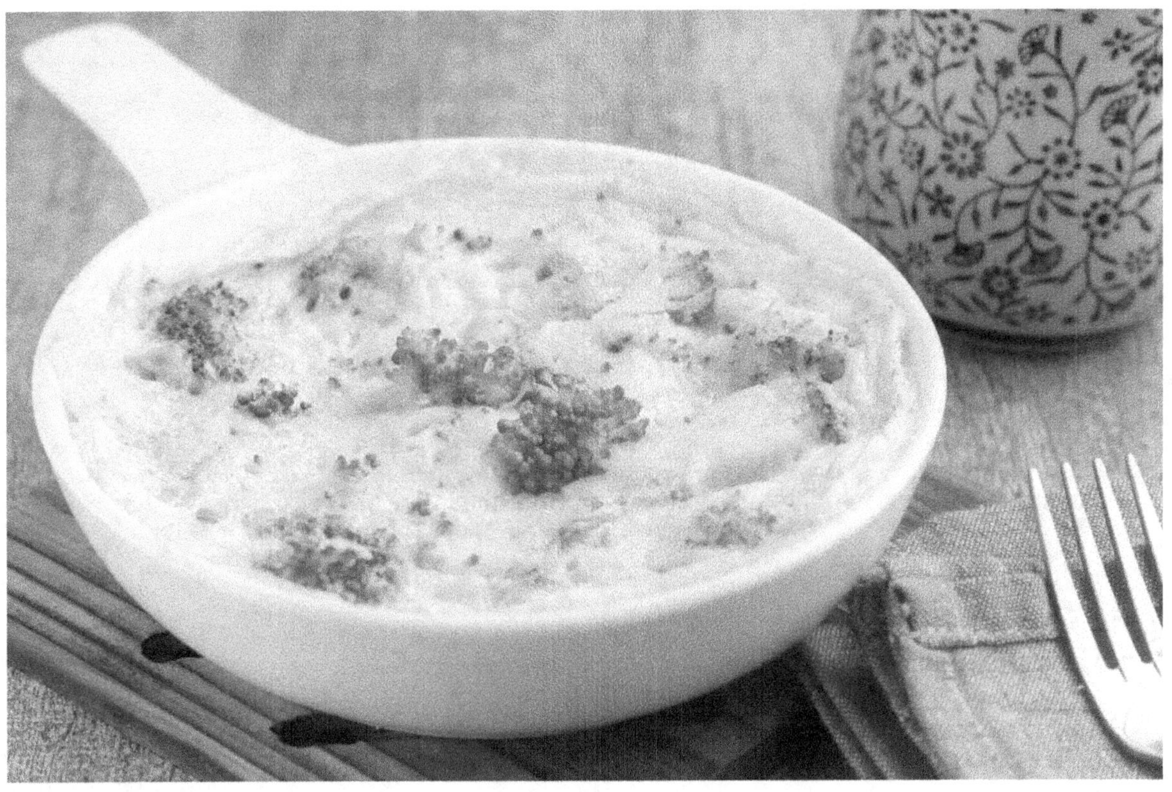

This frittata featured recipe is extraordinarily amazing and stands out as the best of the breakfast recipe you can ever imagine of tasting. Enjoy!

Servings: 2

Cooking time: 45 mins

Ingredients:

- 2 oz. spinach, fresh
- 1½ oz. dried bacon
- 2 eggs
- 1½ oz. shredded cheese
- ¼ c. heavy whipped cream
- ½ tbsp. butter
- Salt and pepper

Instructions:

1. Preheat your oven to 360°F and grease a baking dish.

2. Melt the butter in a skillet and cook the bacon until crispy.

3. Stir in the spinach, then put aside.

4. Beat the eggs with the cream, then pour into your prepared dish.

5. Stir in the bacon and spinach.

6. Cook in your oven for thirty minutes.

7. Serve.

Keto-Friendly Oatmeal

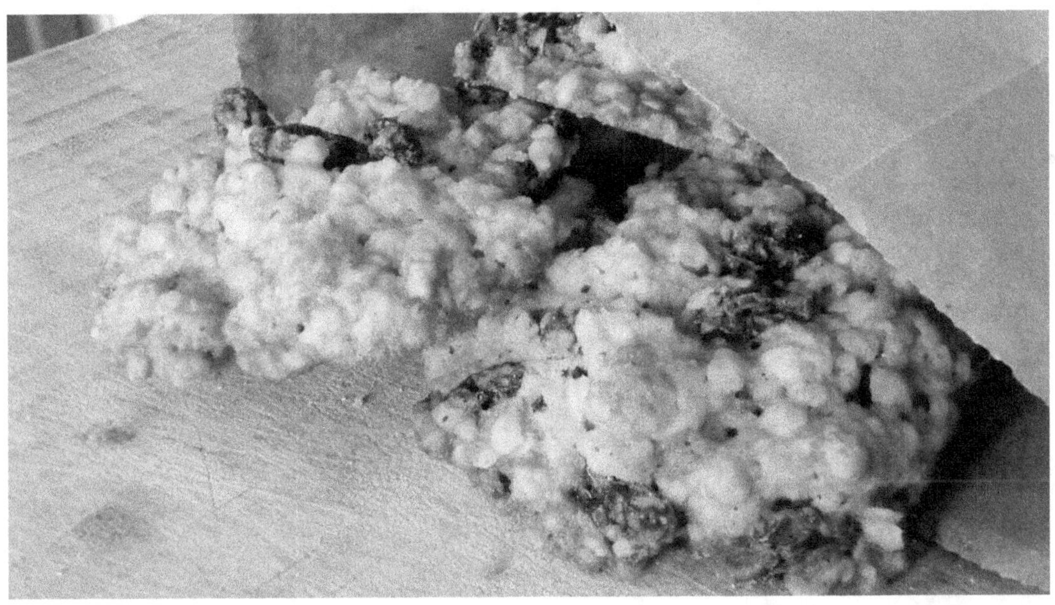

It is a quite easy recipe that you can opt to prepare for your family. The recipe is packed with ingredients that are essential for your health. Enjoy!

Servings: 2

Cooking time: 20 mins

Ingredients:

- 2 tbsps. sunflower seeds
- 2 tbsps. flaxseeds
- 2 tbsps. chia seeds
- 2 c. coconut milk
- 2 pinches salt

Instructions:

1. Chuck everything into a saucepan and mix together.

2. Bring to the boil, then simmer for about seven minutes.

Baked Eggs and Beef

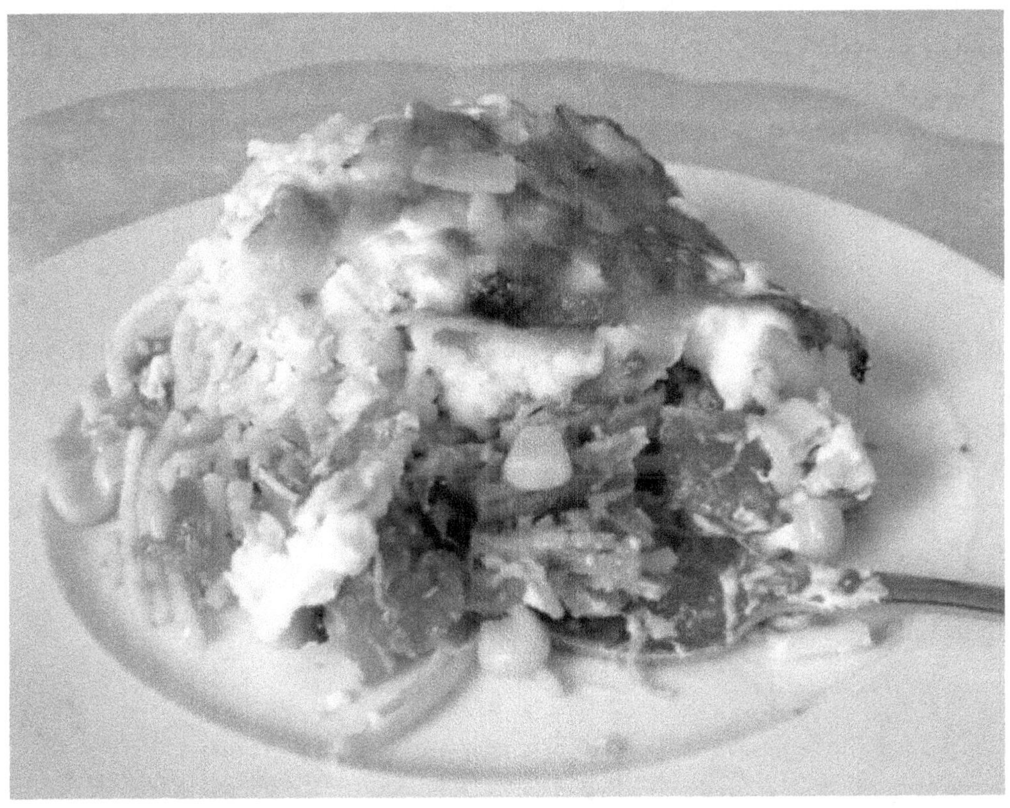

The delicious combination of baked eggs and beef sounds amazing. Of course, it is a perfectly amazing combination. Enjoy.

Servings: 2

Cooking time: 10 mins

Ingredients:

- 2 eggs
- 2 oz. shredded cheddar cheese
- 3 oz. beef, cooked and ground

Instructions:

1. Preheat your oven to 390° and grease a baking dish.

2. Spread your ground beef in the baking dish, making two holes into which you crack the eggs.

3. Sprinkle with cheese, then pop into the oven.

4. Cook for around twenty minutes.

5. Wrap in foil and keep in the fridge for up to two days.

Sausage Sandwich

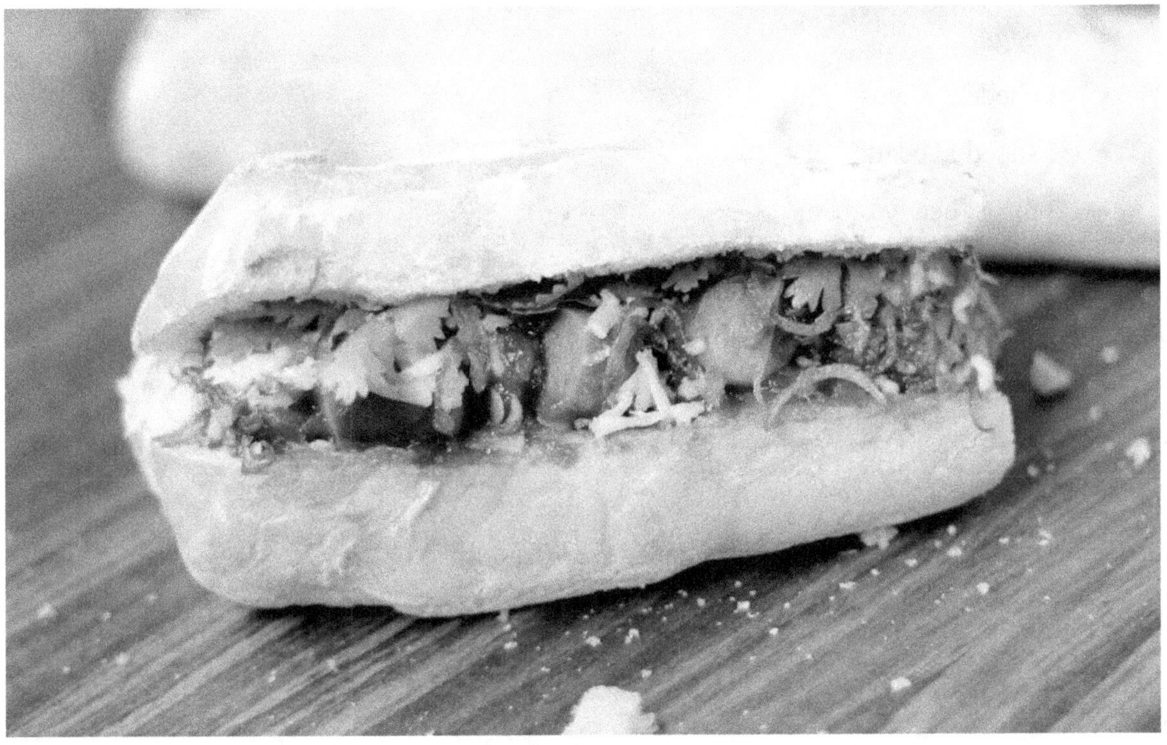

Take your time and prepare the sausage sandwich wonderfully. You are assured to enjoy with your family.

Servings: 3

Cooking time: 20 minutes

Ingredients:

- 6 sausage patties, frozen
- 6 eggs
- 3 cheddar slices
- 1 sliced avocado
- 2 tbsps. heavy cream
- 1 tbsp. butter, melted
- 1 pinch red pepper flakes
- Black pepper and salt

Instructions:

1. Heat sausage patties according to package instructions.

2. Meanwhile, mix eggs, heavy cream, pepper flakes and a generous sprinkle of salt and black pepper in a bowl.

3. Divide the egg mix into thirds and pour the first cup into the skillet. Top with a slice of cheese and cook for 1 minute. Roll up the two sides of the egg into the center to cover the cheese. Transfer to a plate. Do this with the remaining egg mixture.

4. Insert each egg between two sausage patties and serve with avocado.

Breakfast Pancakes

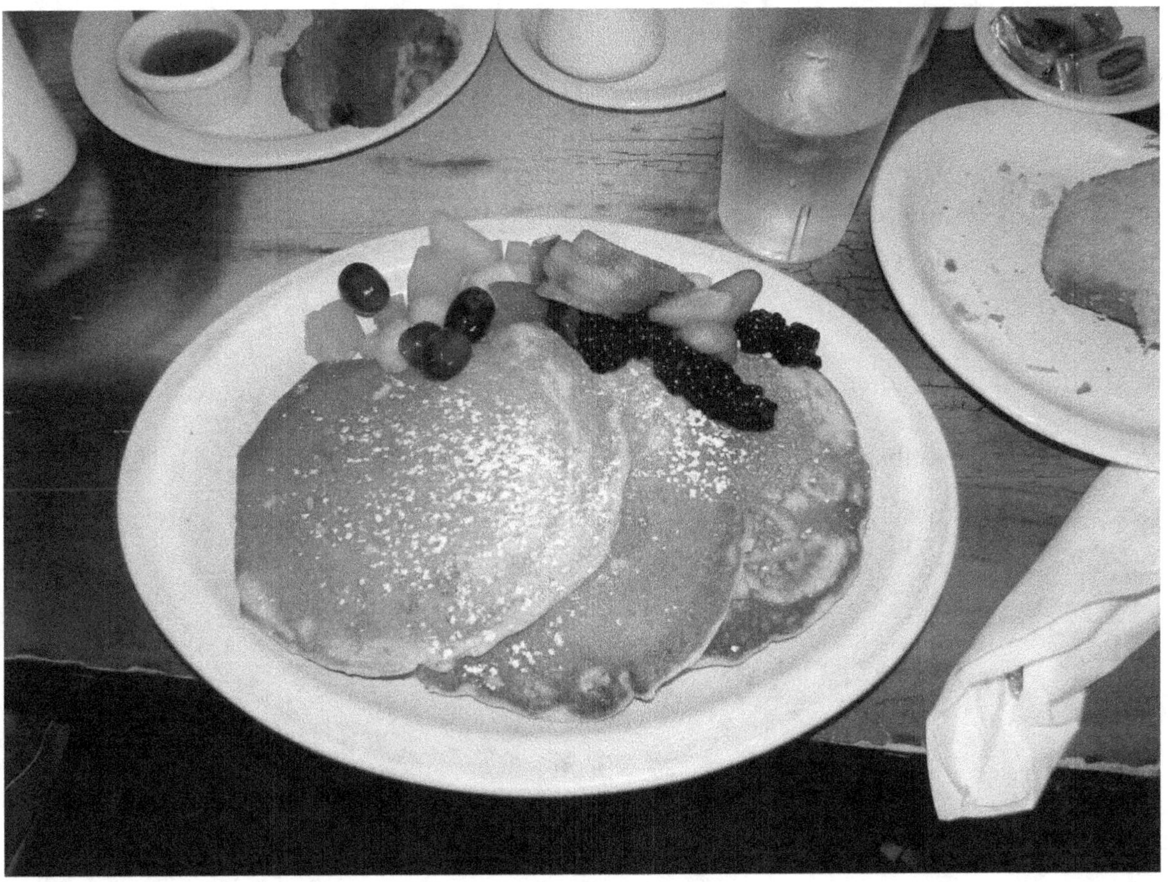

The pancakes are quite thick and spongy. You will love them when served along with one of your favorite foods. Enjoy.

Cooking time: 15 minutes

Servings: 10

Ingredients:

- 4 eggs
- ½ c. almond flour
- 4 oz. cream cheese, softened
- butter
- 1 tsp. lemon zest

Instructions:

1. Combine all ingredients except butter in a bowl.

2. Cook about 3 tablespoons of the batter in 1 tablespoon melted butter over medium heat, for 2 minutes. Set aside in a plate. Do this with the remaining batter and serve topped with butter.

Cheesy Muffins

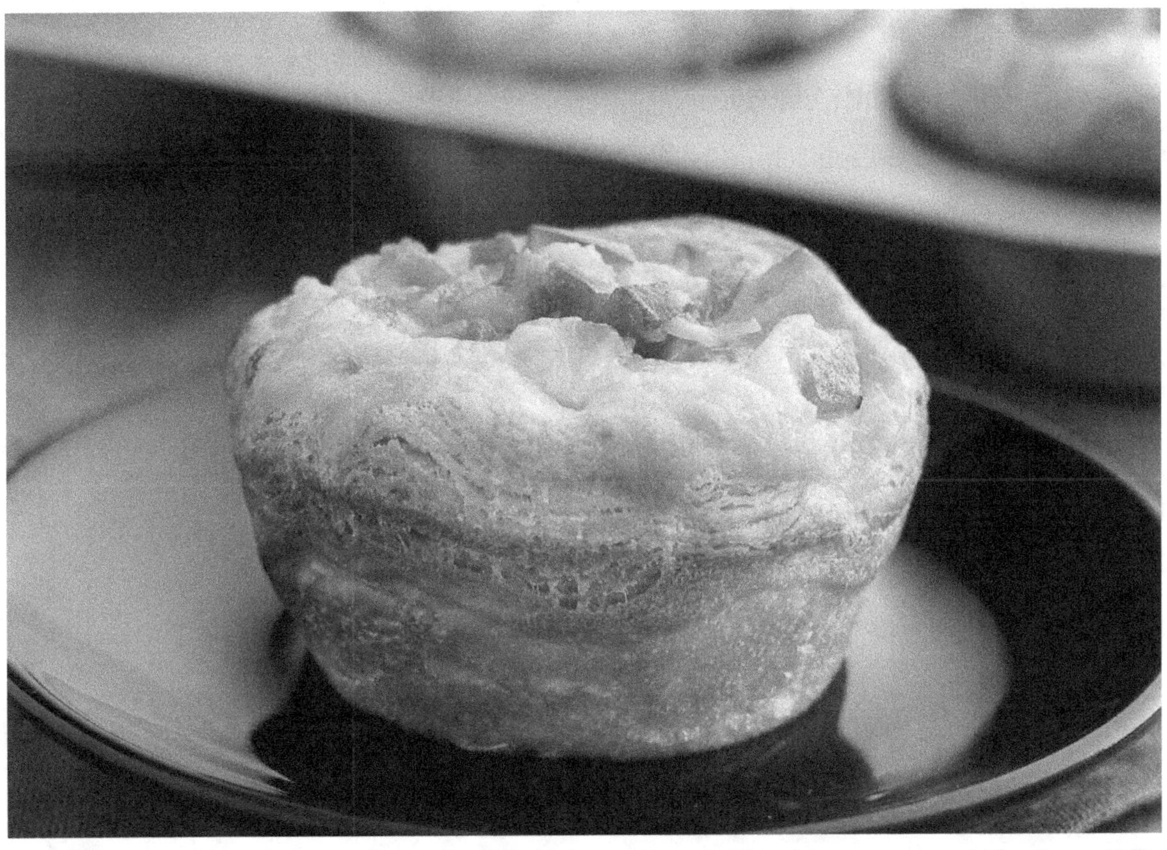

The cheesy muffins will disappear in seconds. They are sweet and delicious! Prepare them and enjoy it!

Cooking time: 25 minutes

Servings: 12

Ingredients:

- 2 lbs. ground pork
- 12 eggs
- 1 c. white cheddar, shredded
- 2 ½ c. chopped spinach
- 1 tbsp. chives, chopped
- 1 tbsp. chopped thyme
- 2 minced garlic cloves
- ½ tsp. ground cumin
- ½ tsp. paprika
- Black pepper
- 1 tsp. salt

Instructions:

1. Preheat the oven to 400°F.

2. Mix together pork, thyme, garlic, cumin, paprika, salt and pepper in a bowl.

3. Use a 12-cup muffin tin and place a small handful of the pork mixture in each cup. Press the sides of each to create a cup shape.

4. Top cups evenly with spinach and cheese, then crack an egg into each cup.

5. Sprinkle with salt and pepper.

6. Bake for 25 minutes. Top with chives before serving.

Almond Protein Shake

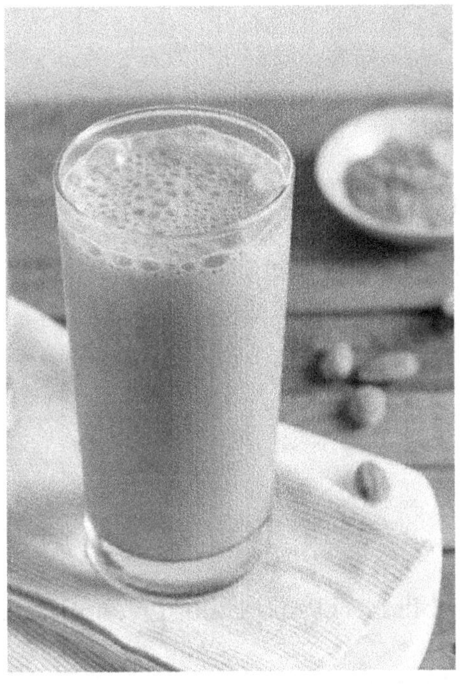

The Almond Protein Shake has a unique delicious taste that will leave you yearning for more and more. Enjoy every moment as you get in touch with the meal.

Servings: 1

Cooking time: 10 minutes

Ingredients:

- ¾ c. almond milk
- 2 tbsps. almond butter
- ½ tbsp. vanilla extract
- ½ c. ice
- 2 tbsps. cocoa powder, unsweetened
- 3 tbsps. sugar substitute (Keto friendly)
- 2 tbsps. hemp seed
- 1 tbsp. chia seeds
- 1 pinch salt

Instructions:

1. Set all ingredients in your blender. Process until well blended.

2. Serve in a glass with any topping of choice.

Mexican Scrambled Eggs

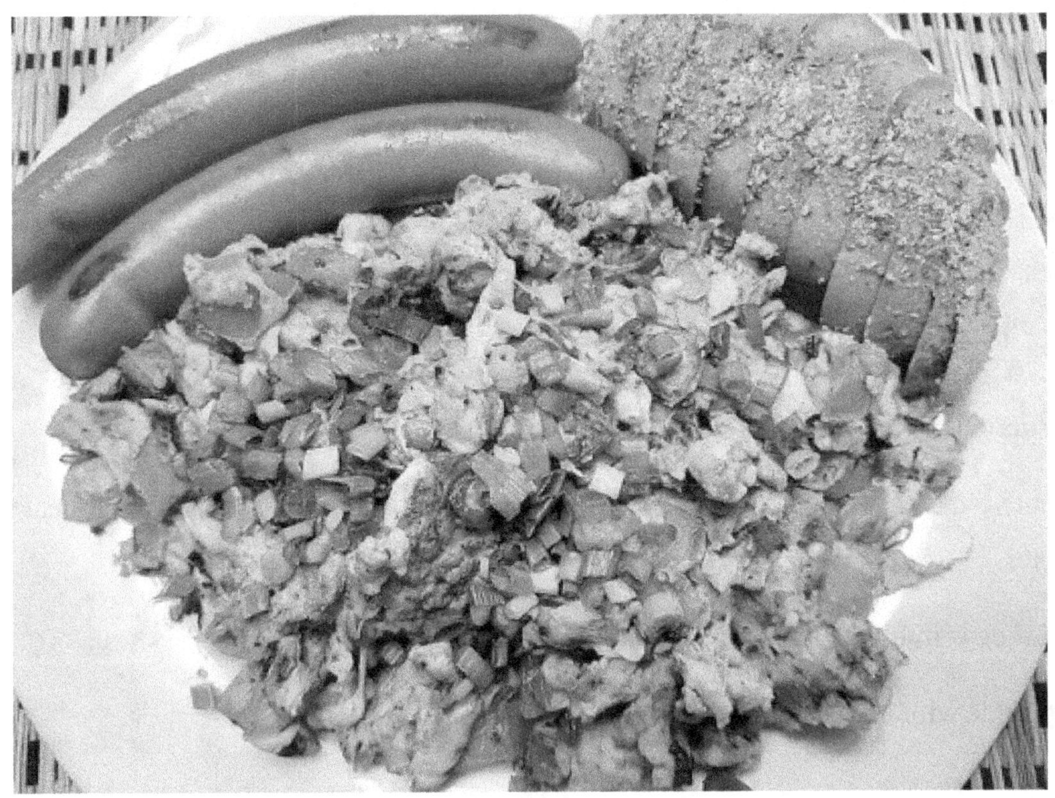

You need the Scrambled eggs to be your default breakfast meal, especially on weekends? Try the preparation and enjoy the perfect moments with your family.

Cooking time: 6 minutes

Servings: 4

Ingredients:

- 6 eggs, beaten
- 3 oz. shredded cheese
- 1 chopped tomato
- 1 oz. butter
- 2 pickled jalapeños, chopped
- 1 chopped scallion
- pepper and salt

Instructions:

1. Sauté tomatoes, jalapeños and scallions in melted butter over medium-high heat for 4 minutes.

2. Pour eggs into the pan and scramble for 2 minutes.

3. Sprinkle with cheese, pepper and salt before serving.

Mushroom Omelet

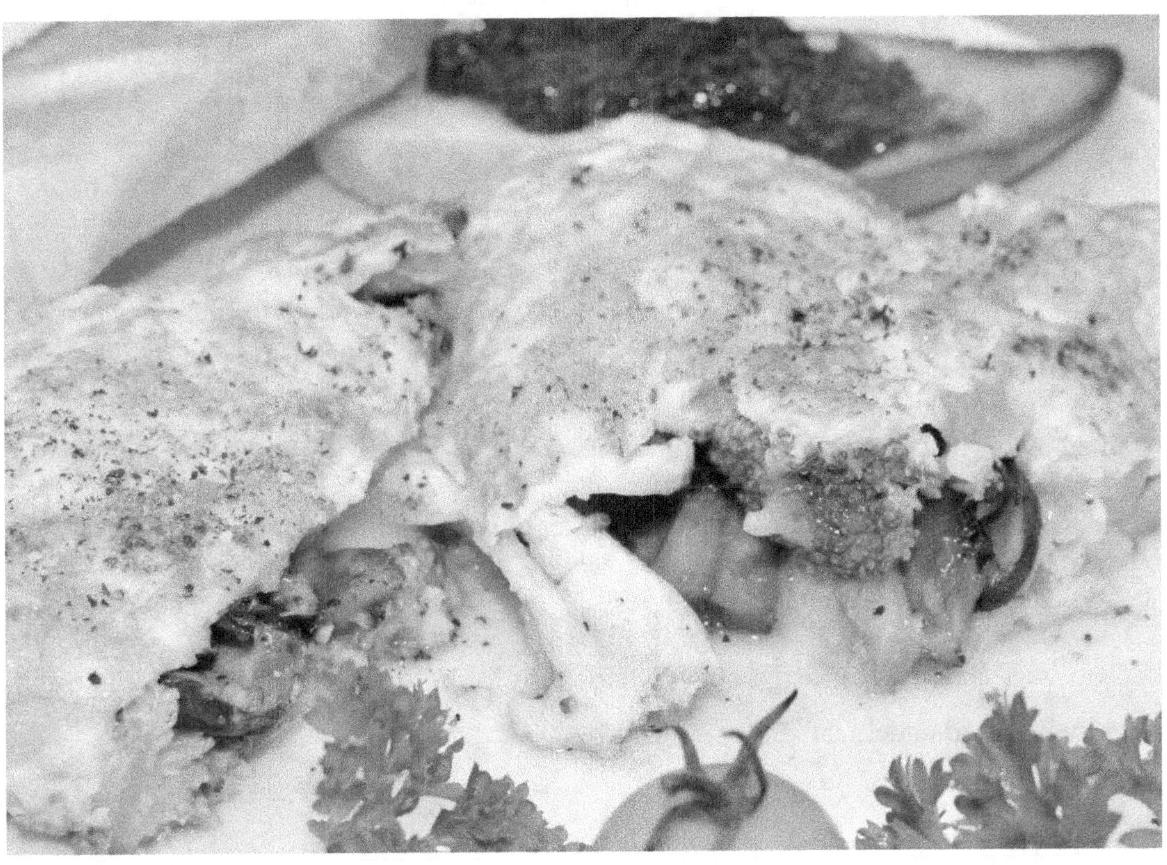

For a breakfast classic, the mushroom omelet is quick and easy to make. Along with other fillings, you will get the best from the omelet.

Cooking time: 25 minutes

Servings: 1

Ingredients:

- 4 sliced mushrooms
- 3 eggs
- 1 oz. shredded cheese
- 1 oz. butter
- ¼ yellow onion, chopped
- pepper and salt

Instructions:

1. In a bowl, whisk eggs with pepper and salt.

2. Sauté mushrooms and onions in melted butter over medium heat until tender.

3. Add the egg mixture around the veggies.

4. Top with cheese when eggs begin to cook. Fold the omelet in half, then cook until slightly browned underneath.

Hash Browns

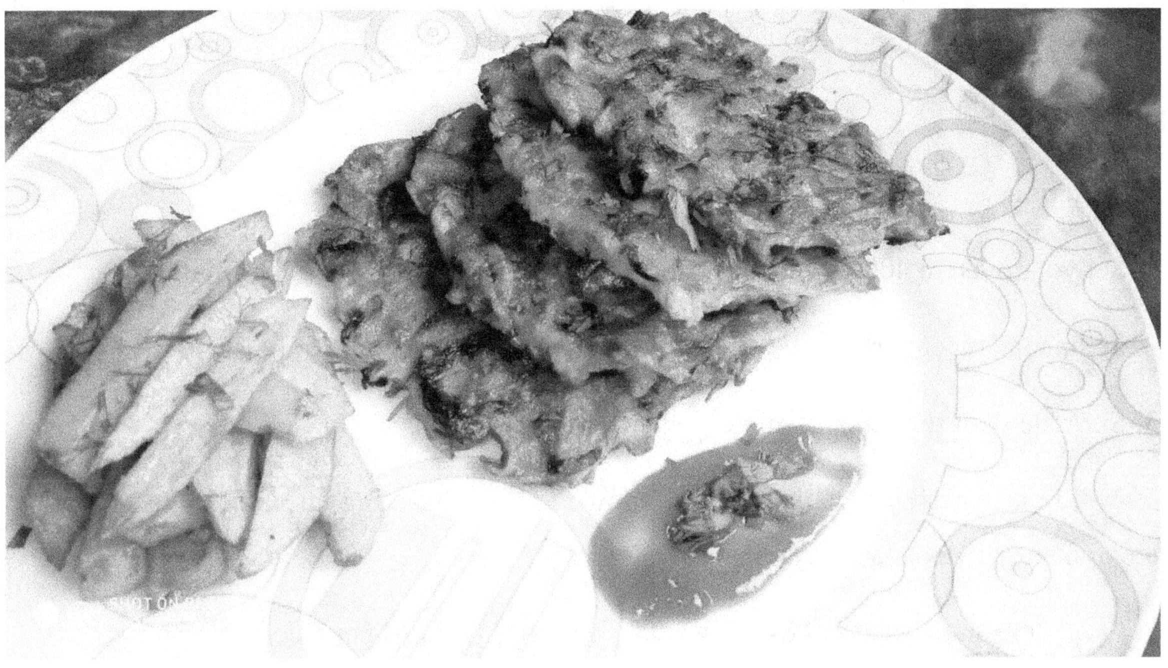

Hash browns are the simplest and most popular meals that easy to follow the recipe. Try them to enjoy a wonderful breakfast.

Cooking time: 64 minutes

Servings: 5

Ingredients:

- 1 whole spaghetti squash, halved and deseeded
- 3 tbsps. avocado oil
- sea salt

Instructions:

1. Set your oven to 400°F and bake the squash, cut sides down, for 50 minutes.

2. Scrape the inner parts of the squash into a bowl using a spoon and discard the skin.

3. Sprinkle with sea salt and mix together.

4. Mold the squash into balls and press down to form hash brown patties. Do away with any moisture in excess using paper towels.

5. Fry patties in avocado oil over medium heat for 7 minutes per side.

Taco Skillet

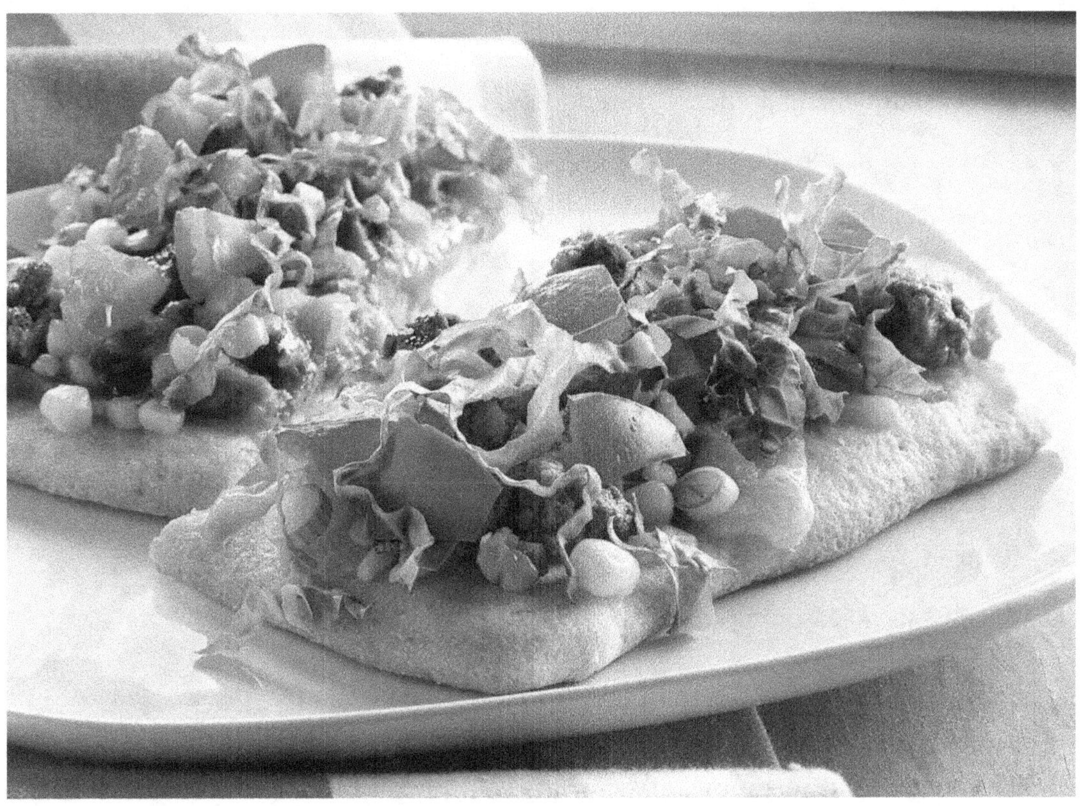

An easy, mouth-watering, and delicious meal to cook, especially for your kids. The perfect combination of ingredients sounds amazing. Try this delicacy and keep yourself strong.

Cooking time: 45 minutes

Servings: 6

Ingredients:

- 1 lb. ground beef
- 10 eggs
- 1 ½ c. sharp cheddar cheese, shredded, divided
- 1 diced Roma tomato
- ¼ c. sliced black olives
- 1 chopped avocado
- ¼ c. heavy cream
- ¼ c. sour cream
- ¼ c. salsa
- ⅔ c. water
- 2 sliced green onions
- 4 tbsps. taco seasoning

Instructions:

1. Adjust your heat to medium high. Set a skillet in place and cook ground beef until browned. Drain the excess fat using a paper towel.

2. Season beef with the taco seasoning, add water. Stir and simmer on low heat for 5 minutes. Transfer half of the cooked beef to a plate.

3. Whisk eggs in a bowl. Add 1 cup of cheddar cheese and heavy cream.

4. Preheat the oven to 375°F.

5. Top the skillet meat with the egg mixture and stir to combine.

6. Bake for 30 minutes and serve topped with the remaining ground beef, tomato, ½ cup cheddar cheese, avocado, olives, green onions, salsa and sour cream.

Porridge

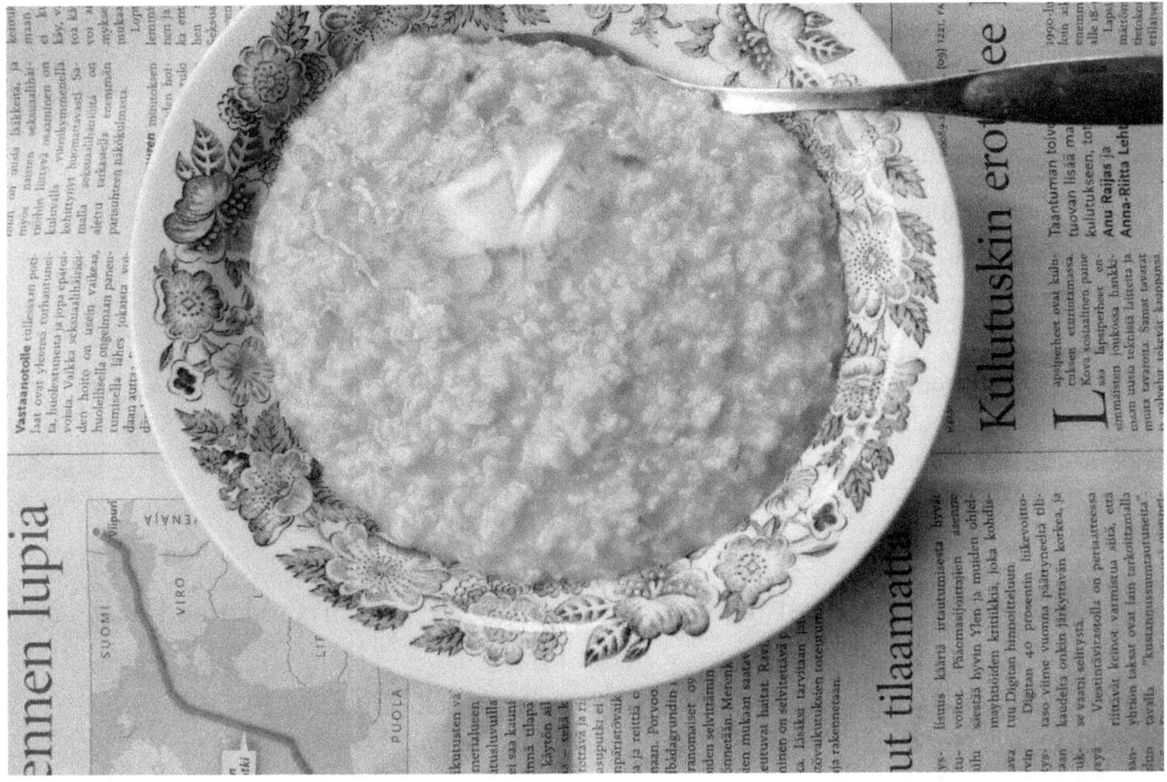

Porridge is a wonderful dish that is common to almost everyone. The meal can be prepared in different ways, and at the end, you will have different but unique tastes. Enjoy!

Cooking time: 4 minutes

Servings: 1

Ingredients:

- 1 tbsp. golden flaxseed meal
- ½ tsp. vanilla extract
- ½ c. water
- 2 tbsps. almond flour
- 2 tbsps. shredded coconut, unsweetened
- 2 tbsps. hemp hearts
- 1 tbsp. chia seeds
- ¼ tsp. sweetener of choice
- 1 pinch salt

Instructions:

1. Using a saucepan, mix all ingredients with the exception of vanilla and cook for 5 minutes, stirring frequently, over low heat.

2. Add vanilla and stir.

Radishes and Corned Beef Hash

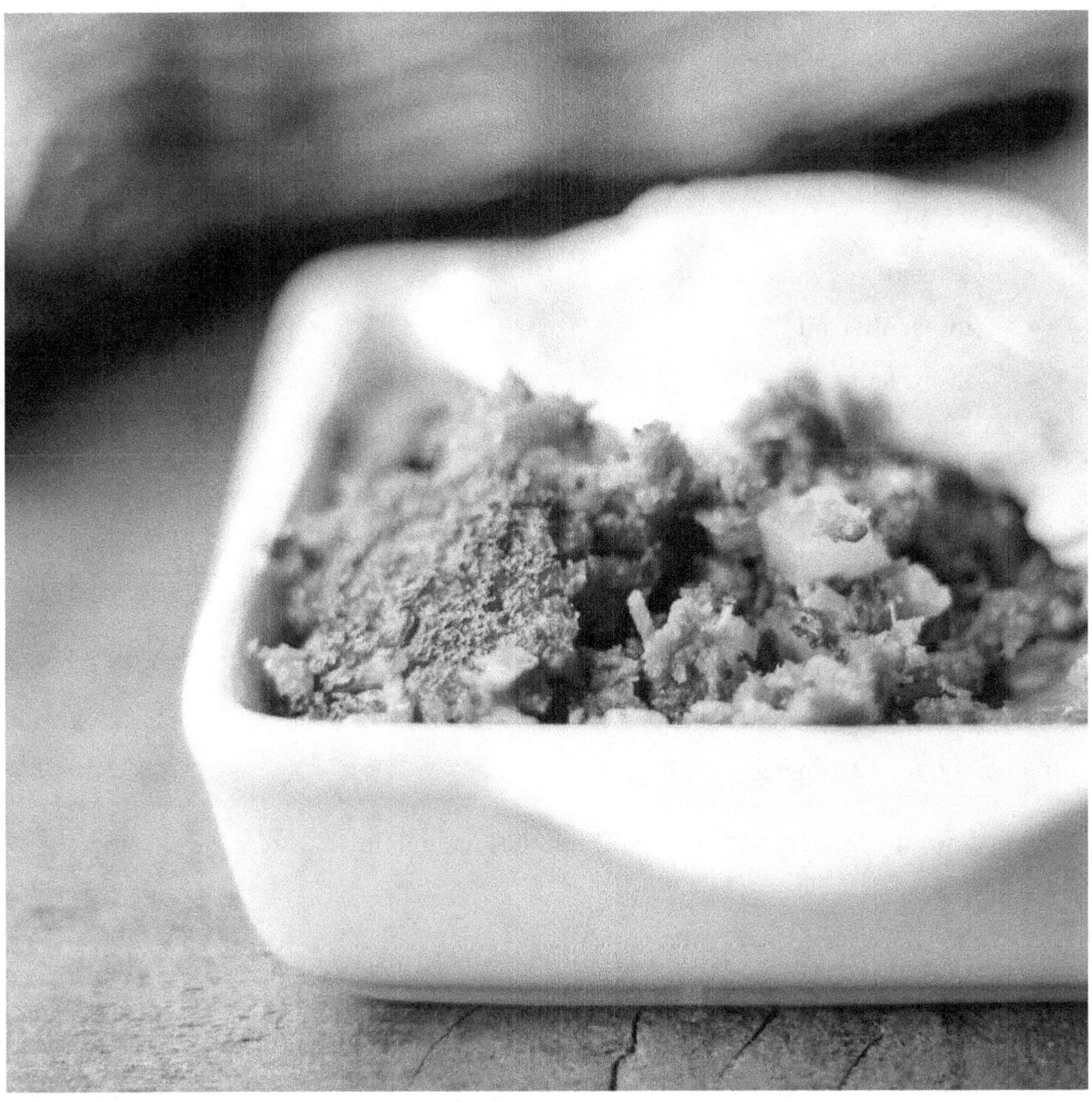

It's awesome to have a taste of the radishes that have been specially combined with corned beef hash and other ingredients. Enjoy.

Cooking time: 18 minutes

Servings: 4

Ingredients:

- 1 c. diced radishes
- 12 oz. corned beef
- 1 tbsp. olive oil
- 1 sliced avocado
- ½ c. whole-egg mayonnaise
- 2 tbsps. olive oil
- 2 tbsps. lemon juice
- 1 bunch chives, chopped
- 1 garlic clove

Instructions:

1. Sauté radishes, onions, pepper and salt in olive oil over medium heat, for 5 minutes.

2. Add corned beef, oregano and garlic and cook over medium-low heat, stirring infrequently, for 10 minutes.

3. Press down the mixture and cook for 3 minutes on high heat.

Dark Thick Choco Shake

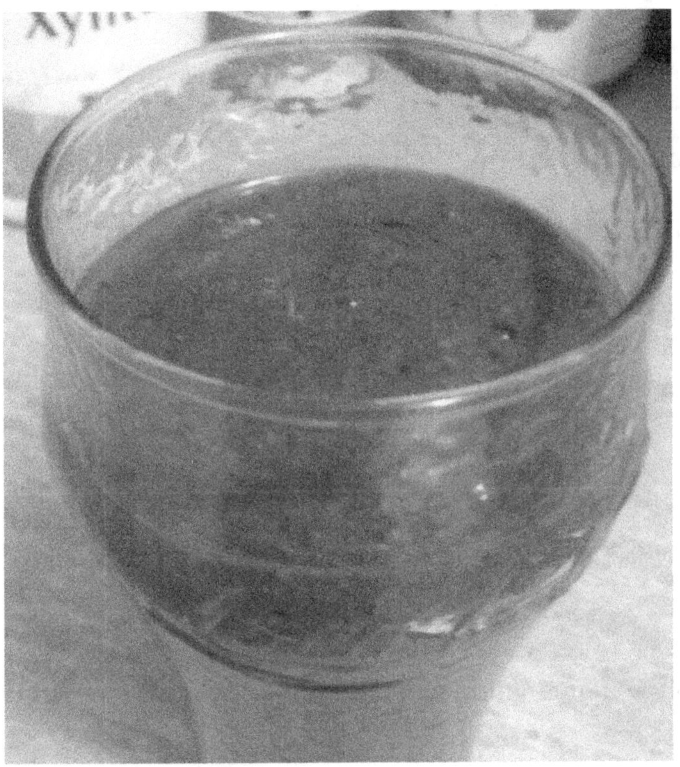

For a meal that will be favorite and friendly for your kids, the dark thick coco shake will do better. It is a mouth-watering meal that provides all the desired sweetness. Enjoy!

Cooking time: 10 minutes

Servings: 2

Ingredients:

- 1 oz. dark chocolate, low carb
- ½ avocado
- 1 tbsp. cacao powder
- ½ c. chilled coconut cream
- ½ c. almond milk
- 1 c. ice
- 2 tbsps. hulled hemp seeds
- 2 tbsps. powdered erythritol

Instructions:

1. Blend cacao powder, hemp seeds and erythritol in a high-powered blender until well blended.

2. Set in the rest of the ingredients and pulse well to obtain a smooth mixture.

Main Meal Recipes

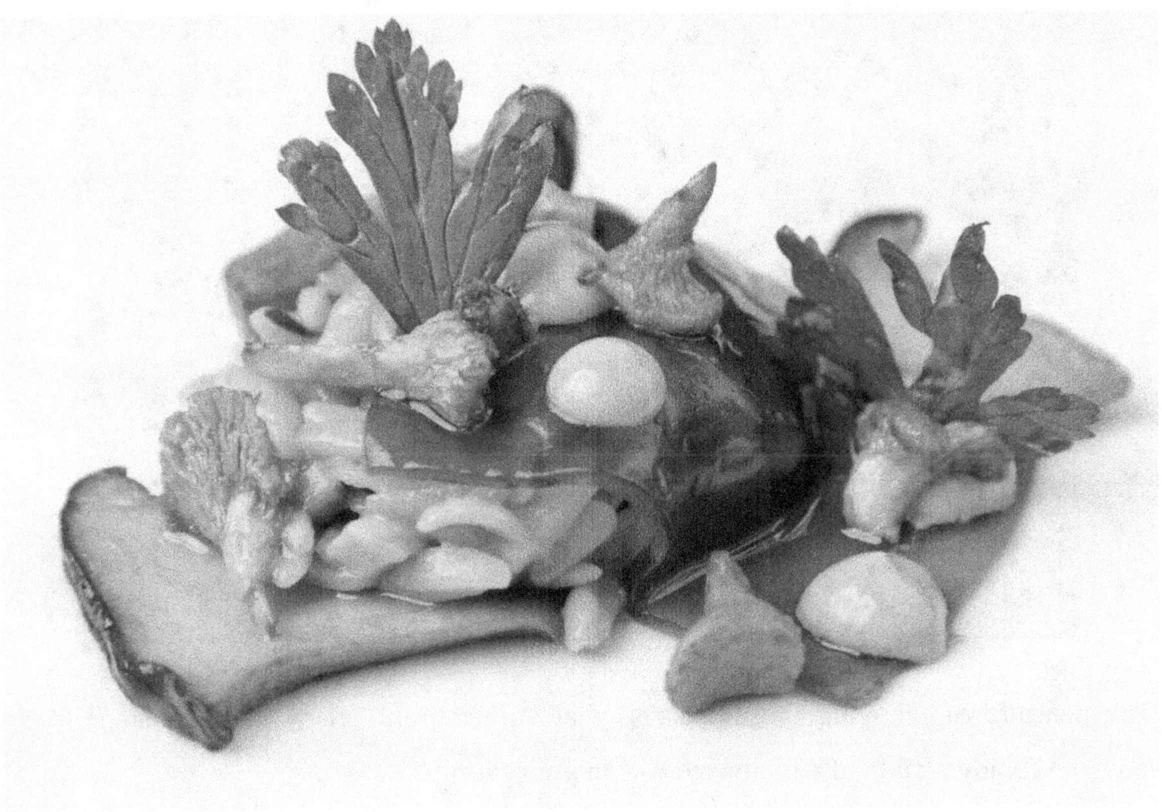

It is so good and wonderful to have a main meal that will strengthen your day and generally take care of your health. The recipes here have been specially chosen to help you cope with the Keto diet and live a healthy life. Each of the recipes has specially chosen ingredients that are essential for your health. Enjoy in every moment of having a taste of these meals.

Crispy Chicken

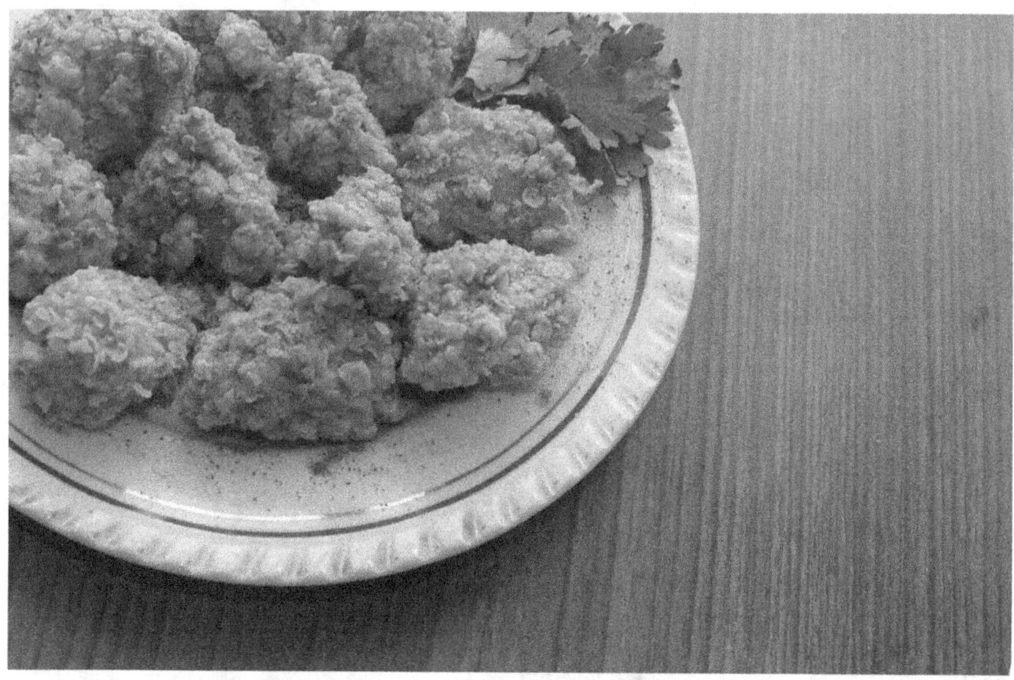

The pleasure of enjoying the sweetness that comes from crispy chicken is perfectly amazing. Enjoy a table of deliciousness with your family.

Servings: 2

Cooking time: 40 mins

Ingredients:

- 2 skinned chicken breasts, boned
- 2tbsps. butter
- ¼ c. sour cream
- ¼tsp. turmeric powder
- Salt and pepper

Instructions:

1. Preheat your oven to 360°F and grease a baking dish.

2. Rub the chicken with the turmeric powder and salt and pepper, then pop into the baking dish.

3. Cook for ten minutes, then serve topped with the sour cream.

4. Serve.

Champagne Salmon

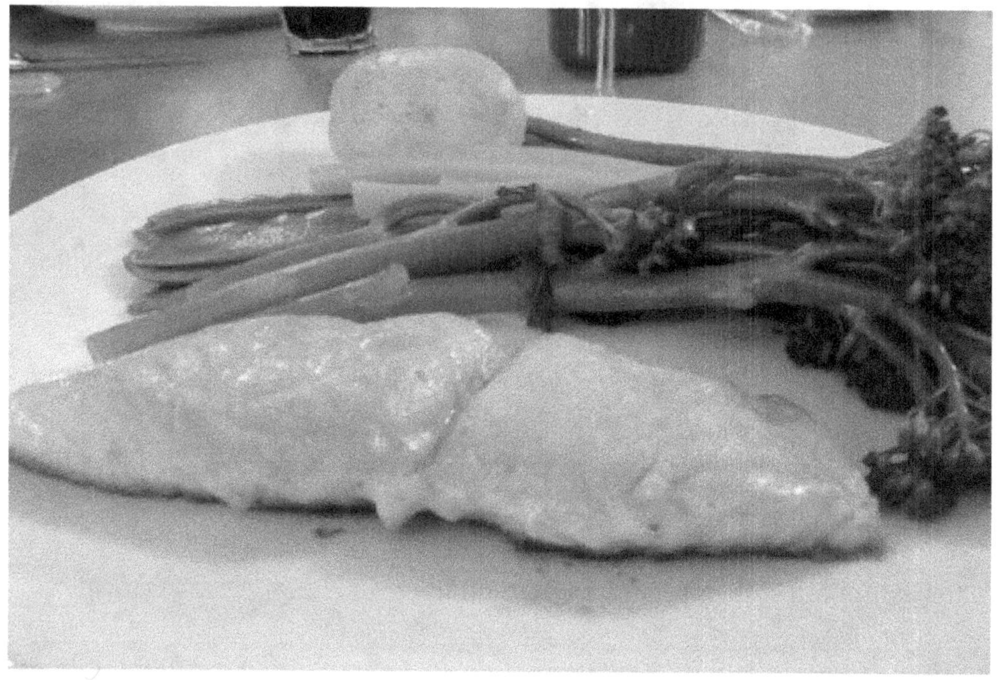

You will love the deliciousness that comes with the preparation of a salmon that has been incorporated with some little champagne. Enjoy!

Servings: 2

Cooking time: 30 mins

Ingredients:

- 2 salmon fillets
- 4 asparagus stalks
- 1tsp. olive oil
- ¼ c. champagne
- ¼ c. butter
- Salt and pepper

Instructions:

1. Preheat your oven to 355°F and grease a baking dish.

2. Mix all the ingredients together well, then pour into the baking dish and pop in the oven.

3. Cook for twenty minutes.

4. Serve immediately or put in airtight containers in the fridge for one day.

Sour and Sweet Fish

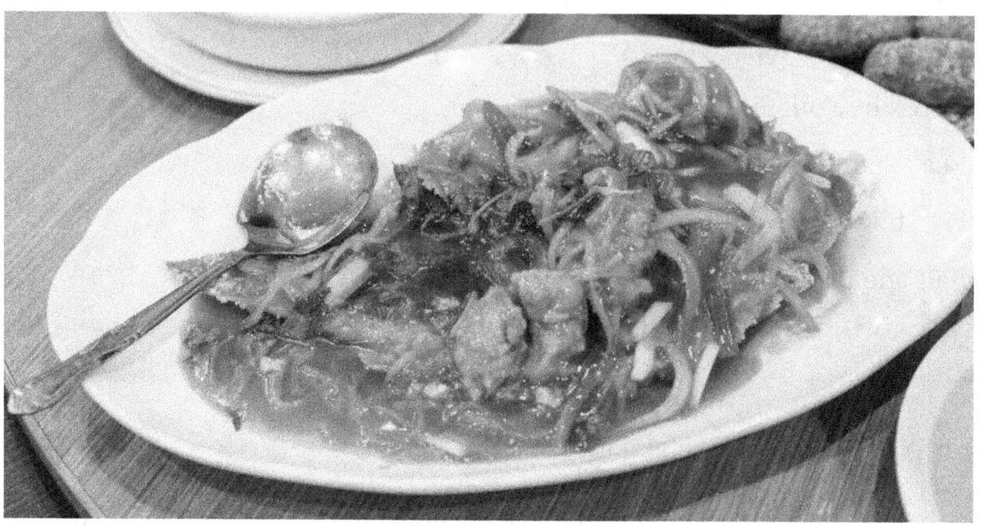

There are multiple ways of preparing fish. The fish meals also range in flavors. This meal is specially prepared and reserved to explore all the sweetness you need.

Servings: 2

Cooking time: 25 mins

Ingredients:

- 1lb. fish chunks
- 2 drops stevia
- 1tbsp. vinegar
- ¼ c. butter, melted
- Salt and pepper

Instructions:

1. Using a skillet, add in butter, then cook the fish for around three minutes.

2. Stir in the stevia, vinegar, and seasoning, then cook for ten minutes, stirring continuously.

3. Serve.

Creamy Chicken and Mushrooms

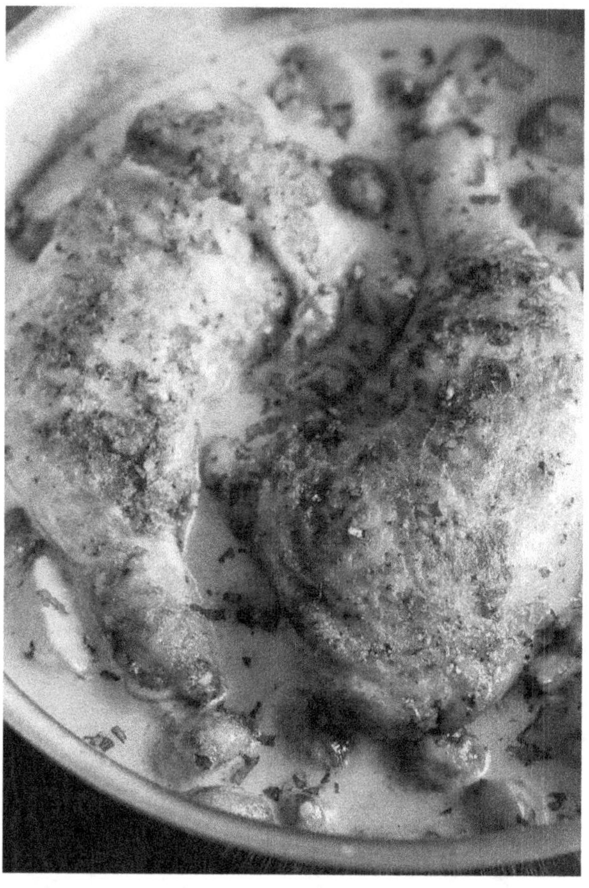

It is a meal to be craved by everyone in your home. The creamy chicken and mushrooms will give you a perfect moment to remain cool and refreshed.

Servings: 2

Cooking time: 25 mins

Ingredients:

- ½lb. chicken breasts
- ¼ c. mushrooms
- ½ onion, chopped
- 1tbsp. butter, melted
- ¼ c. sour cream

Instructions:

1. Using a skillet, add in butter and cook the onions and mushrooms for five minutes.

2. Add the chicken, and season with salt. Cover, and cook for another five minutes.

3. Stir in the sour cream and cook for another three minutes.

4. Serve.

Paprika Shrimp

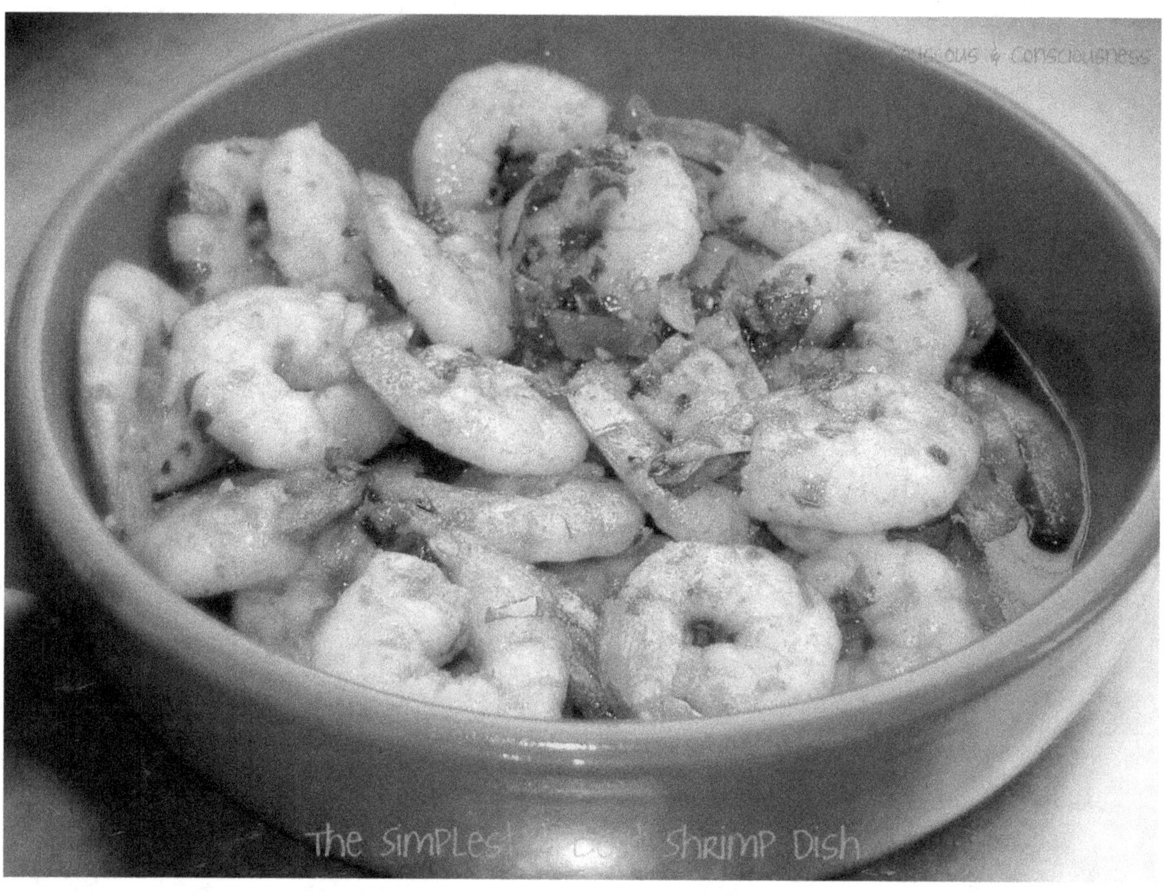

The preparation of shrimps differs in a number of ways. A taste of a shrimp prepared in this manner will be a great privilege. Enjoy.

Servings: 2

Cooking time: 30 mins

Ingredients:

- ½ lb. shrimp
- 1/8 c. butter
- ¼ tbsp. smoked paprika
- 1/8 c. sour cream
- Salt and pepper

Instructions:

1. Preheat your oven to 390°F and grease a baking dish.

2. Mix everything together until well combined, then pop into the baking dish.

3. Cook in the oven for around fifteen minutes.

4. Serve.

Cheesy Spinach Chicken

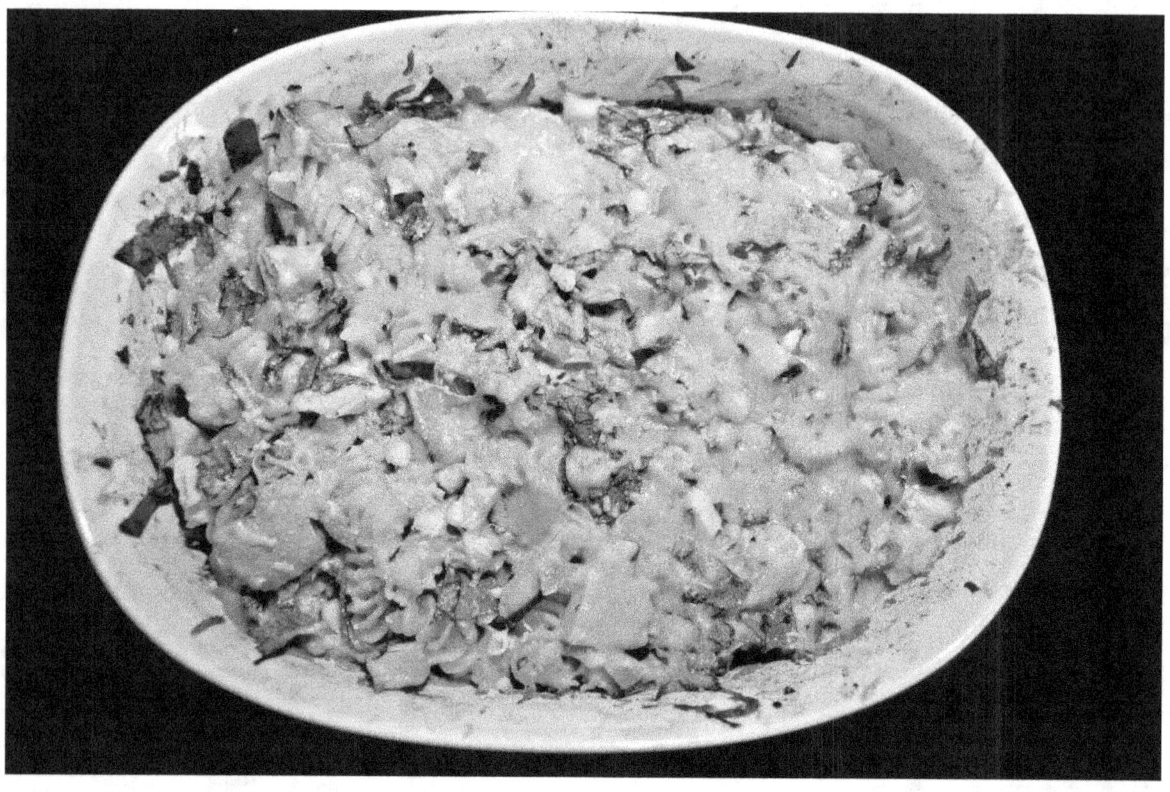

The cheesy spinach chicken will definitely be the family's favorite. It entails simple instructions that make it easy and quick to prepare.

Servings: 2

Cooking time: 20 mins

Ingredients:

- ¾ lb. chicken tenders
- ¼ c. parmesan cheese, shredded
- 10 oz. frozen spinach, chopped
- 2 garlic cloves, minced
- 2tbsps. unsalted butter, divided
- ¼ c. heavy cream
- Salt and pepper

Instructions:

1. Using a skillet, set in half of the butter and melt, then add the chicken with salt and pepper.

2. Cook for three sides per minutes, the reserve.

3. Using a skillet, melt the remaining butter, then add the garlic, heavy cream, cheese, and spinach.

4. Cook for two minutes, then return the chicken to the skillet.

5. Cook for a further five minutes.

6. Serve.

Paprika Prawns

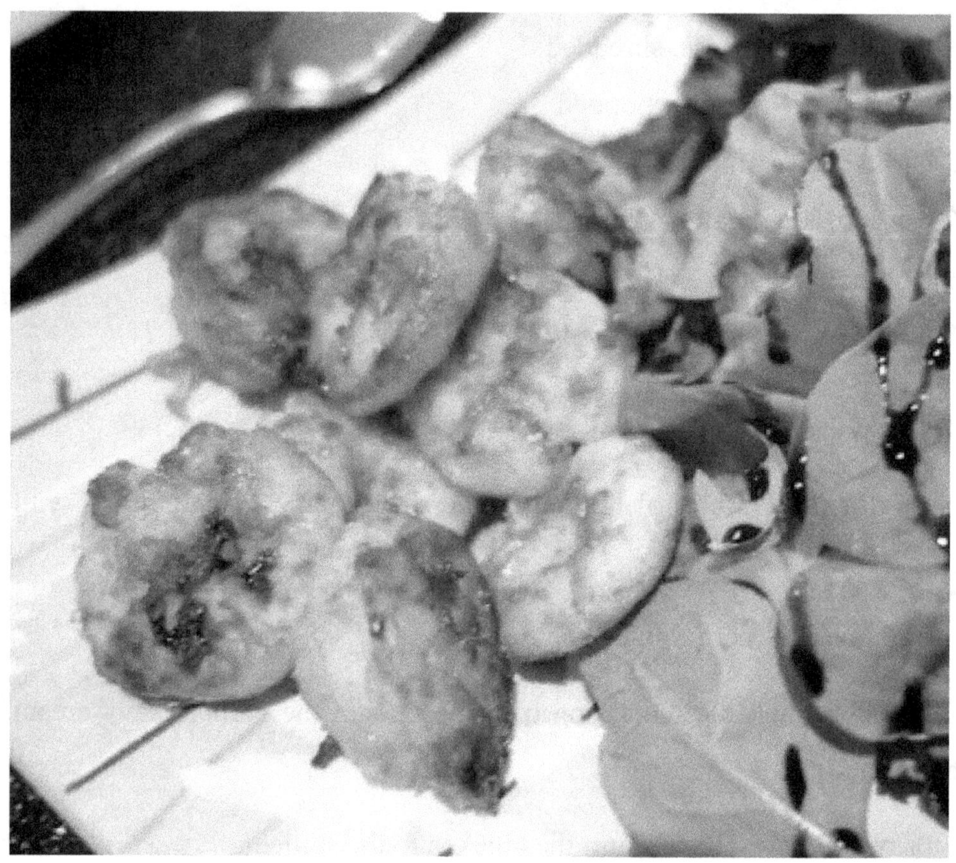

The paprika prawns are specially prepared with not as many ingredients as you would expect. Prawns, paprika, red chili, among others, will give you the flavor you deserve!

Servings: 2

Cooking time: 25 mins

Ingredients:

- ½ lb. deveined prawns, peeled
- ¼ tsp. smoked paprika
- ½ seeded red chili pepper, chopped
- 2 lemongrass stalks
- 6 tbsps. butter

Instructions:

1. Preheat your oven to 390°F and grease a baking dish.

2. In a bowl, stir together the butter, red chili pepper, smoked paprika, and prawns.

3. Leave to marinate for two hours, then thread onto the lemongrass stalks.

4. Cook in the over for fifteen minutes.

5. Serve.

Zucchini-Based Pizza

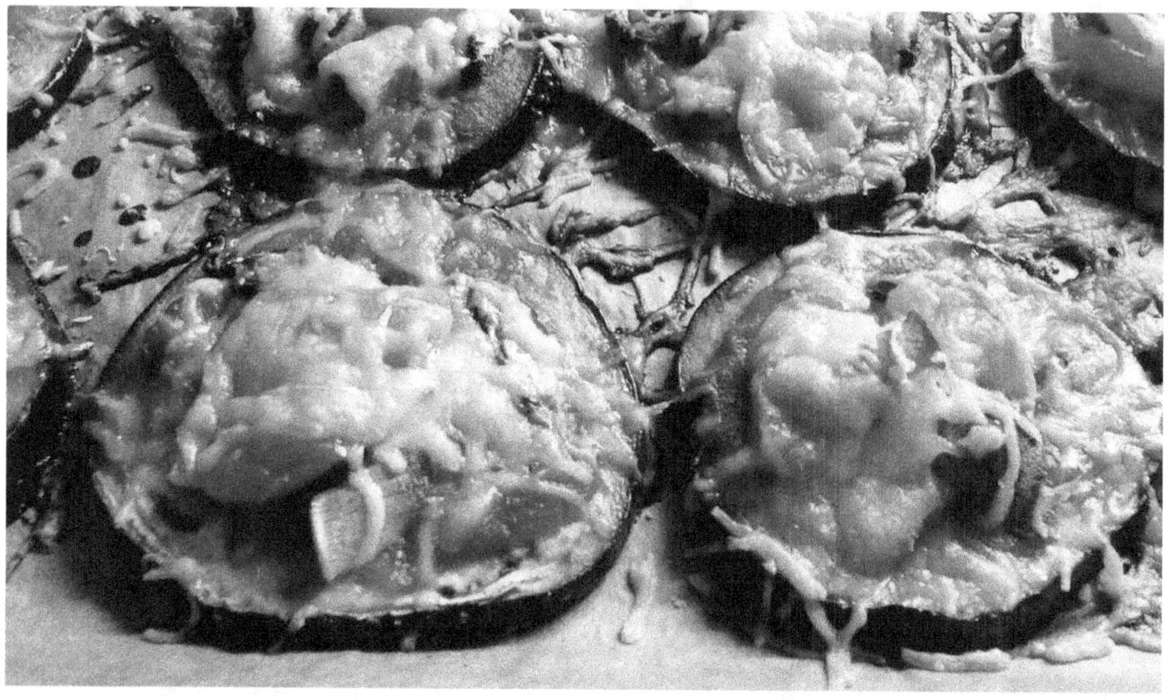

It is a tasty pizza that will satisfy all your cravings for a wonderful meal. Enjoy every minute that comes with having a taste of this pizza.

Servings: 2

Cooking time: 15 mins

Ingredients:

- ½ zucchini, sliced
- Pepperoni slices, for topping
- 1/8 c. spaghetti sauce
- ½ c. shredded mozzarella cheese
- ½ c. cream cheese

Instructions:

1. Set your oven to 350°F and grease a baking dish.

2. Put the zucchini at the bottom of the baking dish, then top with spaghetti sauce.

3. Add the cheese, then the pepperoni, and cook for fifteen minutes.

4. Serve immediately.

Salmon Salad

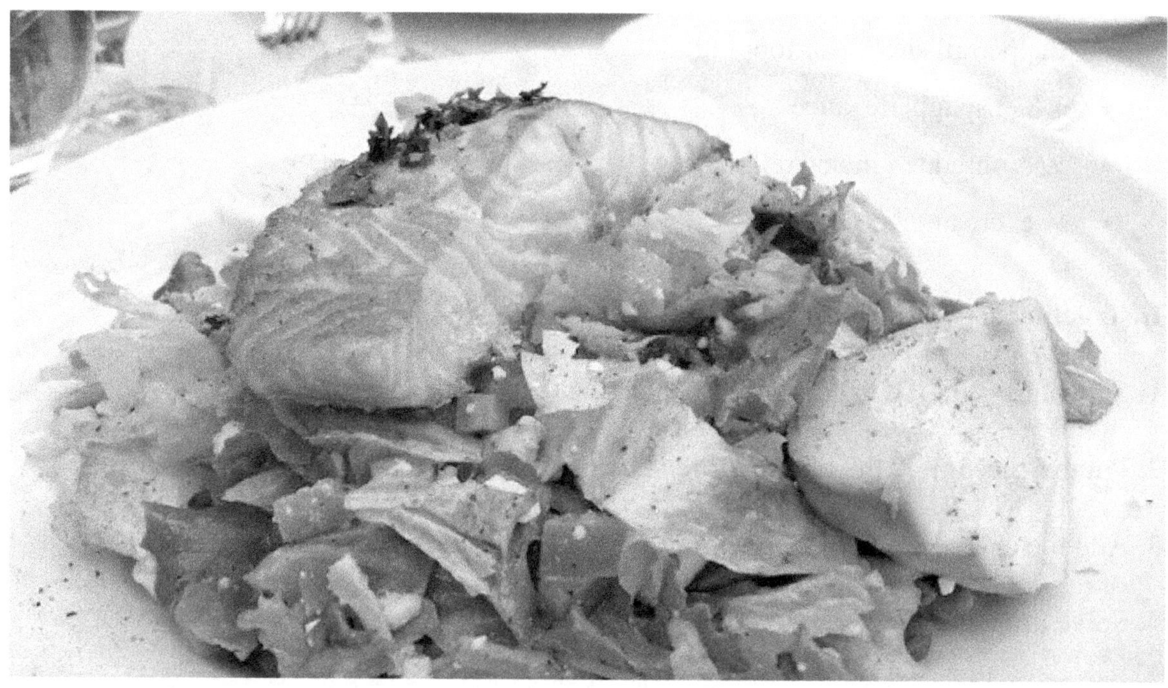

The meal is enriched with all flavors that will give you a perfect touch. Enjoy the sweetness that comes with this salad.

Servings: 2

Cooking time: 15 mins

Ingredients:

- ½ lb. skinless salmon fillet, cut into 4 steaks
- ¼ zucchini, cubed
- ¼ tsp. seeded jalapeño pepper, chopped
- ¼ tbsp. lime juice, fresh
- 1 tbsp. olive oil, divided
- 4 tbsps. sour cream
- ¼ tbsp. fresh dill, chopped
- Salt and pepper

Instructions:

1. In a skillet, add in oil and heat. Cook the salmon for five minutes per side.

2. Season well, then reserve.

3. Toss the remaining ingredients, the serve topped with the salmon. Serve immediately.

Crab Cakes

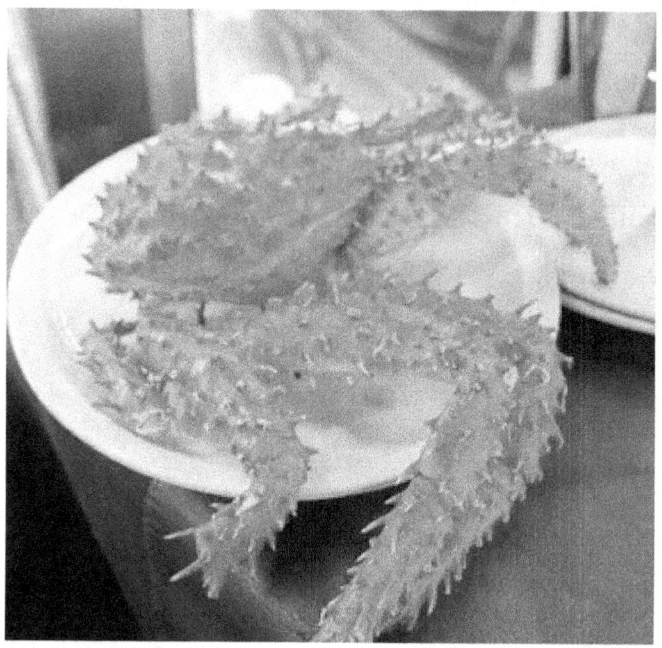

For a more delicate flavor that is regarded to be sweeter than any other meal you can imagine of, the crab cakes are a great deal. Let your family enjoy by preparing such cakes for them.

Servings: 2

Cooking time: 30 mins

Ingredients:

- ½ lb. crabmeat, drained
- 1 tbsp. mayonnaise
- 2 tbsps. coconut flour
- ¼ tsp. green Tabasco sauce
- ½ tsp. yellow mustard
- 1 egg, beaten
- 3 tbsps. butter
- ¾ tbsp. freshly chopped parsley
- Salt and pepper

Instructions:

1. Pop everything but the butter into a bowl and mix well. Shape into patties, then reserve.

2. Melt the butter in a skillet and cook the patties for ten minutes per side.

3. Serve.

Salmon Cakes

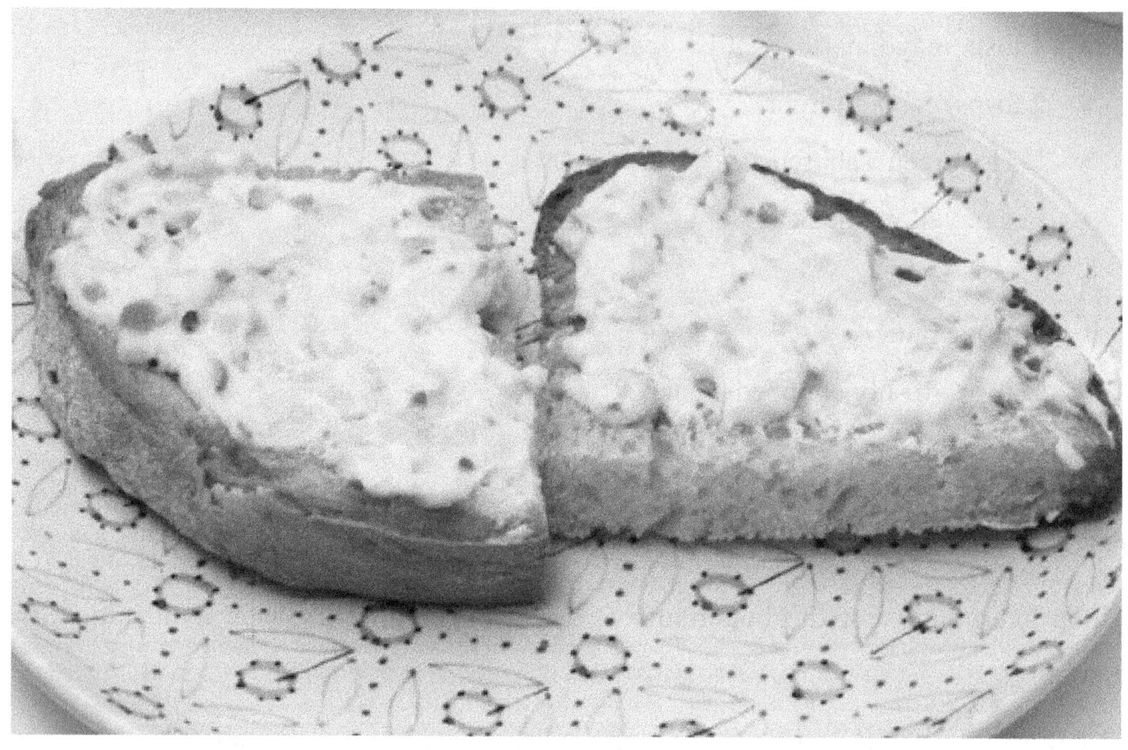

These sweet and tasty salmon cakes don't even need additional sauce. You will enjoy them.

Servings: 2

Cooking time: 20 mins

Ingredients:

- ½ oz. smoked salmon, chopped
- 4 oz. drained pink salmon, deboned
- 1 egg
- 1 tbsp. ranch dressing
- 1/8 c. almond flour
- ½ tbsp. freshly chopped parsley
- ½ tbsp. avocado oil
- ¼ tsp. Cajun seasoning

Instructions:

1. Simply mix everything together well, then shape into patties.

2. Adjust your heat to medium high. Set the patties in a skillet and cook for about three minutes per side.

3. Serve.

Chicken and Vegetables

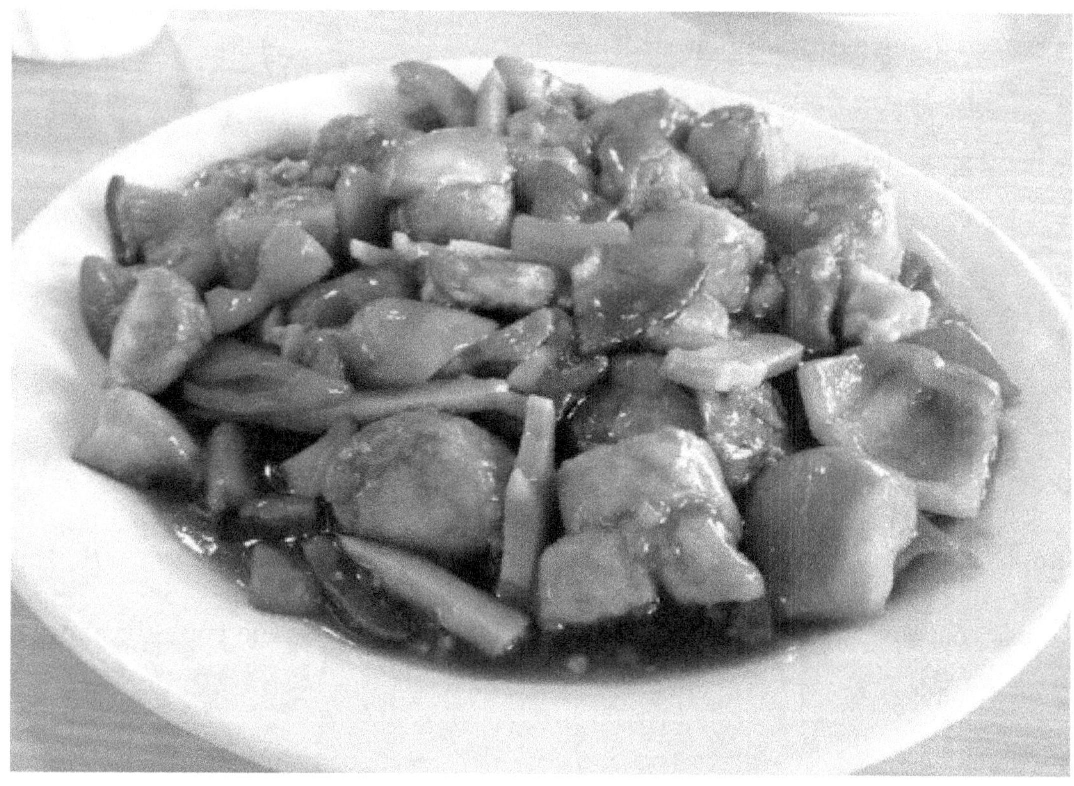

The meal is fresh, sweet, and delicious. A combination of chicken, vegetables, and other ingredients will give that desirable taste.

Servings: 2

Cooking time: 35 mins

Ingredients:

- 6 oz. skinless chicken breasts, boneless sliced
- ½ chopped yellow onion
- ½ chopped zucchini
- ½ c. broccoli florets, fresh
- 1 garlic clove, minced
- ½ tsp. Italian seasoning
- ¼ tsp. paprika
- 1 tbsp. olive oil
- Salt and pepper

Instructions:

1. Set the oven to preheat at 450°F. Using aluminum foil, line a baking dish.

2. Mix all ingredients.

3. Cook for around twenty minutes. Serve immediately or wrap in plastic wrap and store in the fridge for up to five days.

Lemon and Garlic Cauliflower Mash

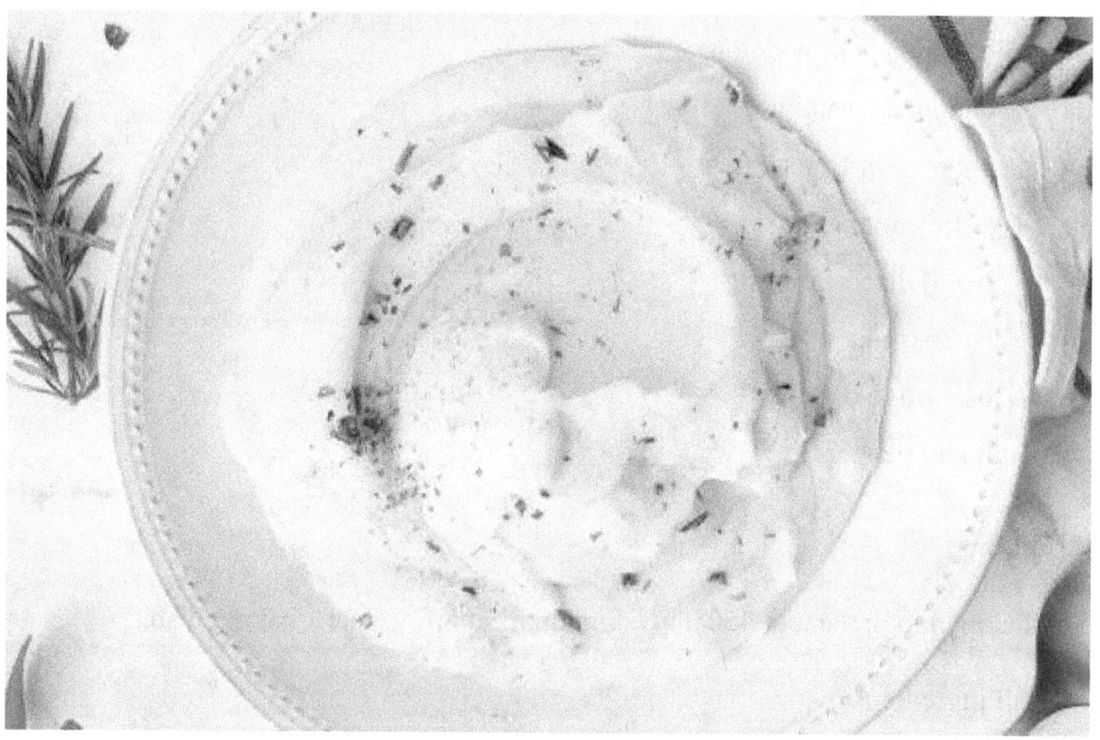

Having a nice meal at the table is everyone's desire. The Lemon and garlic cauliflower mash is a perfect example of foods that will be your family's desire.

Servings: 2

Cooking time: 25 mins

Ingredients:

- 2 c. cauliflower florets
- 1/8 tsp. lemon juice
- ¼ tsp. lemon zest
- ½ tbsp. freshly chopped chives
- ½ clove garlic, peeled
- 1/6 c. avocado mayonnaise
- ½ tbsp. water
- Salt and pepper

Instructions:

1. In a microwave safe bowl, mix the cauliflower, mayonnaise, avocado, water, garlic, and salt and black pepper.

2. Microwave on high for fifteen minutes, then pulse in a food processor.

3. Once smooth, add the lemon juice, zest, and chives, and pulse again until smooth.

4. Serve immediately.

Spaghetti Squash with Cheese and Pesto

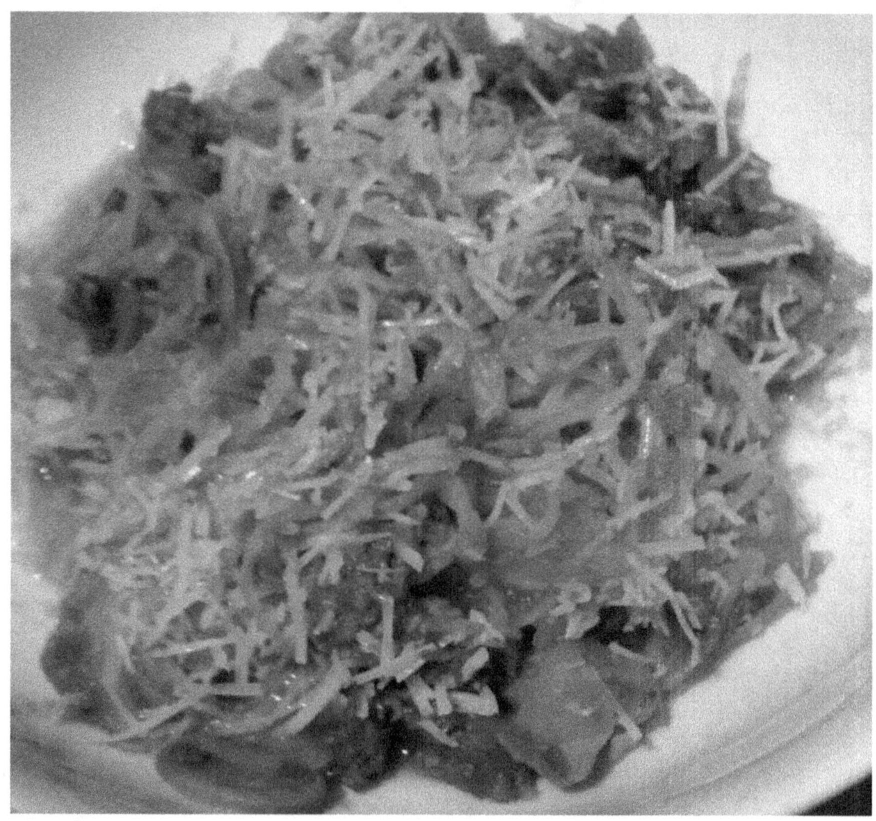

The dish is super-easy in preparation and also wonderful to have on the table. Try it out and enjoy!

Servings: 2

Cooking time: 25 mins

Ingredients:

- 1 c. drained spaghetti squash, cooked
- ½ tbsp. olive oil
- 1/8 c. basil pesto
- ¼ c. whole milk ricotta cheese
- 2 oz. fresh mozzarella cheese, cubed
- Salt and pepper

Instructions:

1. Adjust your oven to 375°F. Grease a casserole dish.

2. In a bowl, mix the squash with the olive oil and salt and pepper.

3. Pop this into the casserole dish, and top with the cheeses.

4. Cook for ten minutes, then serve hot with a drizzle of pesto over the top.

Salmon and Egg Salad

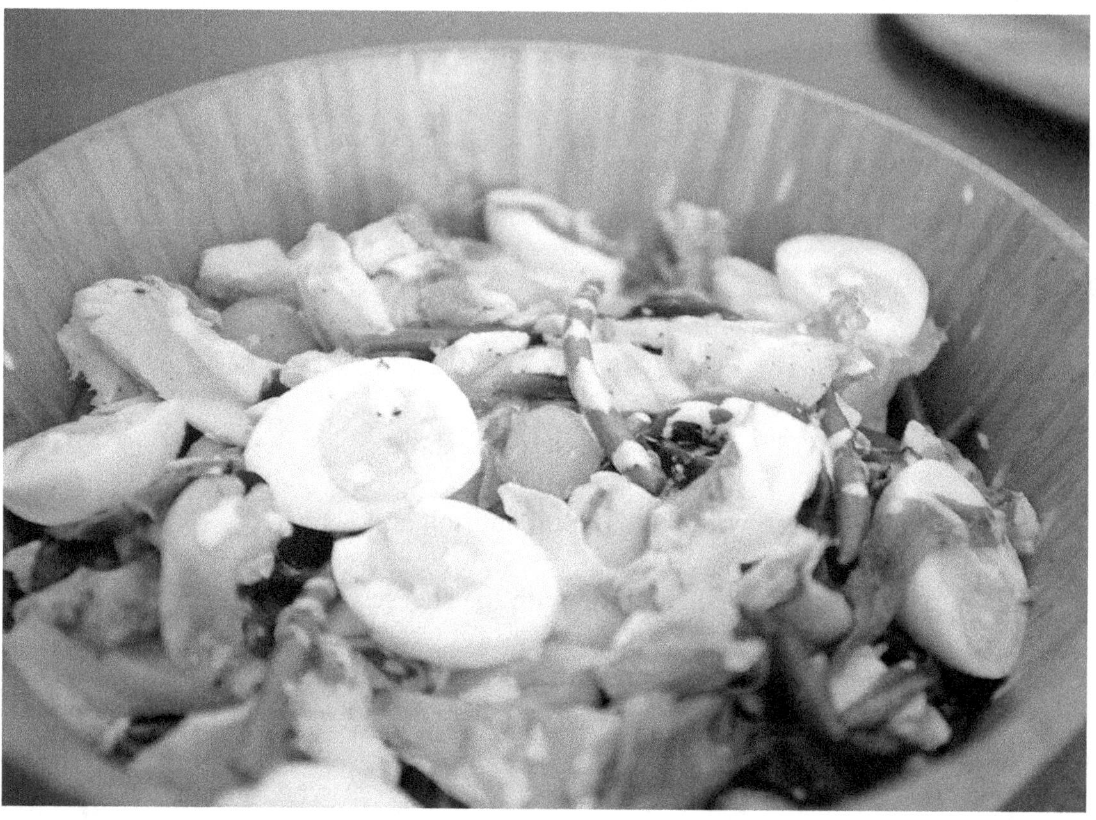

The salad is fresh, vibrant, and fully packed with essential ingredients. Enjoy it.

Servings: 2

Cooking time: 40 mins

Ingredients:

- 6 oz. cooked and chopped salmon
- 4 hard-boiled peeled eggs, cubed
- ¾ c. avocado mayonnaise
- 2 chopped celery stalks
- ½ chopped yellow onion
- 1 tbsp. fresh dill, chopped
- Salt and pepper

Instructions:

1. Using a bowl, set in everything to mix.

2. Use plastic wraps to cover and refrigerate for three hours.

3. Serve immediately or refrigerate for up to three days.

Cheese and Sausage Casserole

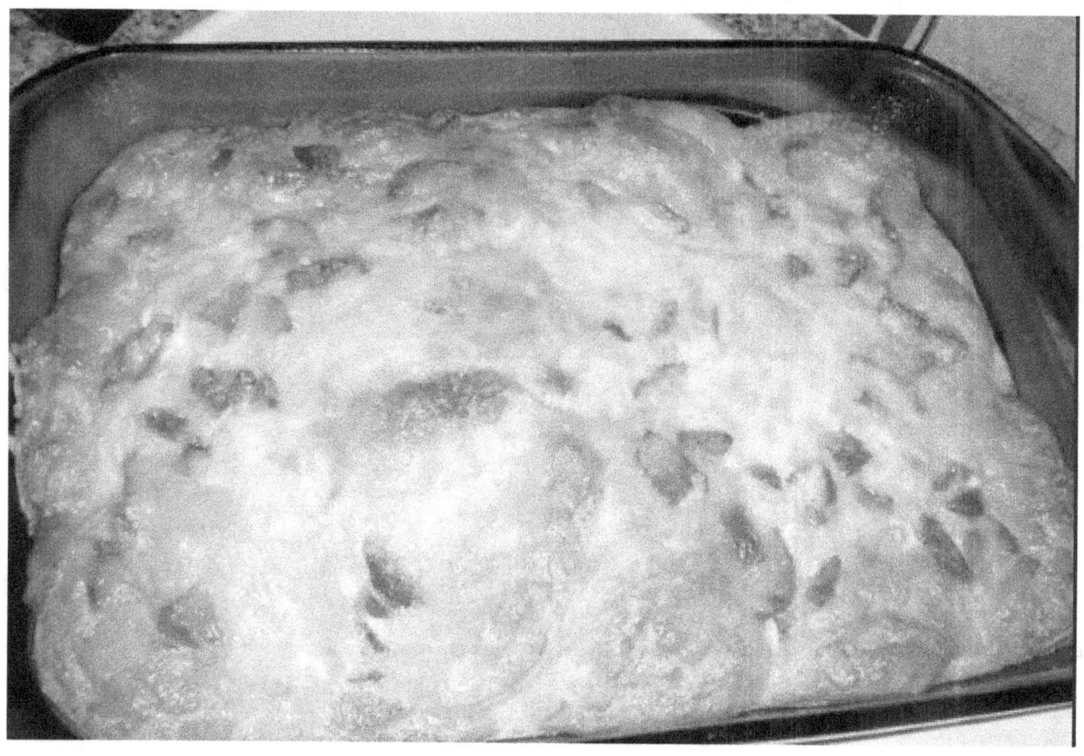

It is a perfect meal to prepare for a good number of people. Showcase your cooking skills by preparing the easy cheese and sausage casserole.

Servings: 2

Cooking time: 46 mins

Ingredients:

- ½ lb. sausages, scrambled
- 4 oz. shredded parmesan cheese
- 4 oz. shredded mozzarella cheese
- 2½ oz. marinara sauce
- ½ tbsp. olive oil

Instructions:

1. Set your oven to 375°F and grease a baking dish with olive oil.

2. Pour in half your sausage, the half the sauce, and half of each cheese.

3. Repeat, and put in the oven for twenty minutes.

4. Serve immediately, or refrigerate for up to two days, and microwave to reheat.

Air Fried Steak

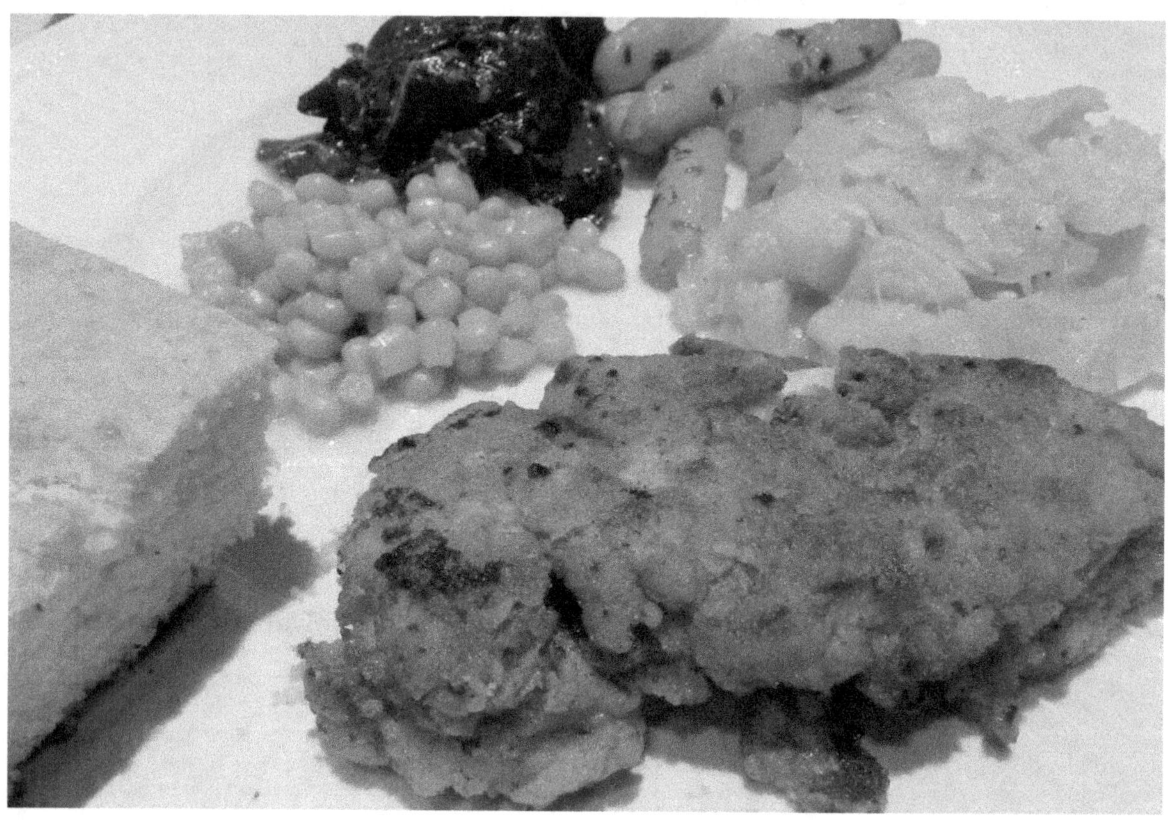

The air-fried steak perfect and easy meal. To those who are likely to prepare it, you are assured of enjoying it as well.

Servings: 2

Cooking time: 15 mins

Ingredients:

- ½ lb. quality cut steaks
- Salt and pepper

Instructions:

1. Preheat your air fryer to 385°F.

2. Rub your steaks all over with salt and pepper.

3. Pop them into the basket of your fryer and cook for fifteen minutes.

4. Serve.

Turkey Breasts in a Garlic Cream Sauce

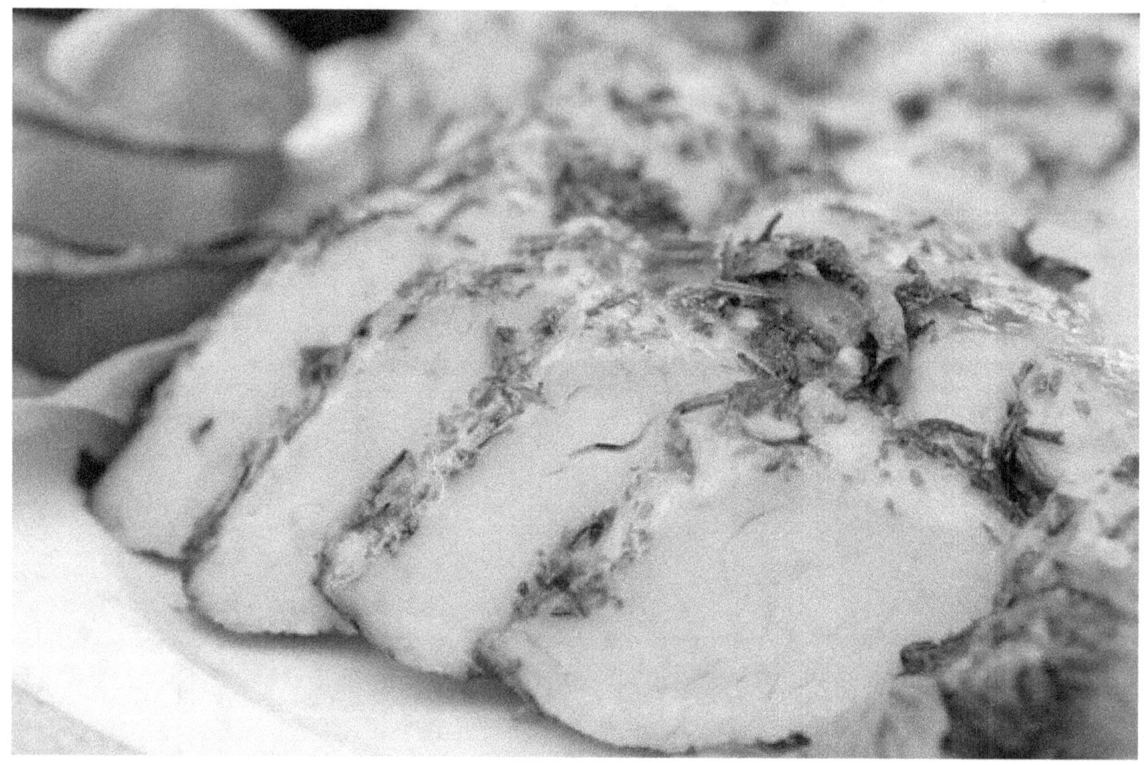

The meal is full of taste, especially when garlic cream sauce is incorporated in it. Other ingredients are also essential in the preparation for the meal.

Servings: 2

Cooking time: 1 hour

Ingredients:

- ¾ lb. turkey breasts
- 2 minced garlic cloves
- ½ c. heavy whipping cream
- ¼ c. sour cream
- ¼ c. butter
- Salt and pepper

Instructions:

1. Preheat your oven to 390°F and grease a baking dish with butter.

2. Rub the turkey breasts all over with the butter, garlic, and salt and pepper, then pop them into the baking dish.

3. Top with the whipping and sour creams, then bake for 45 minutes.

4. Serve.

Tofu Provincial

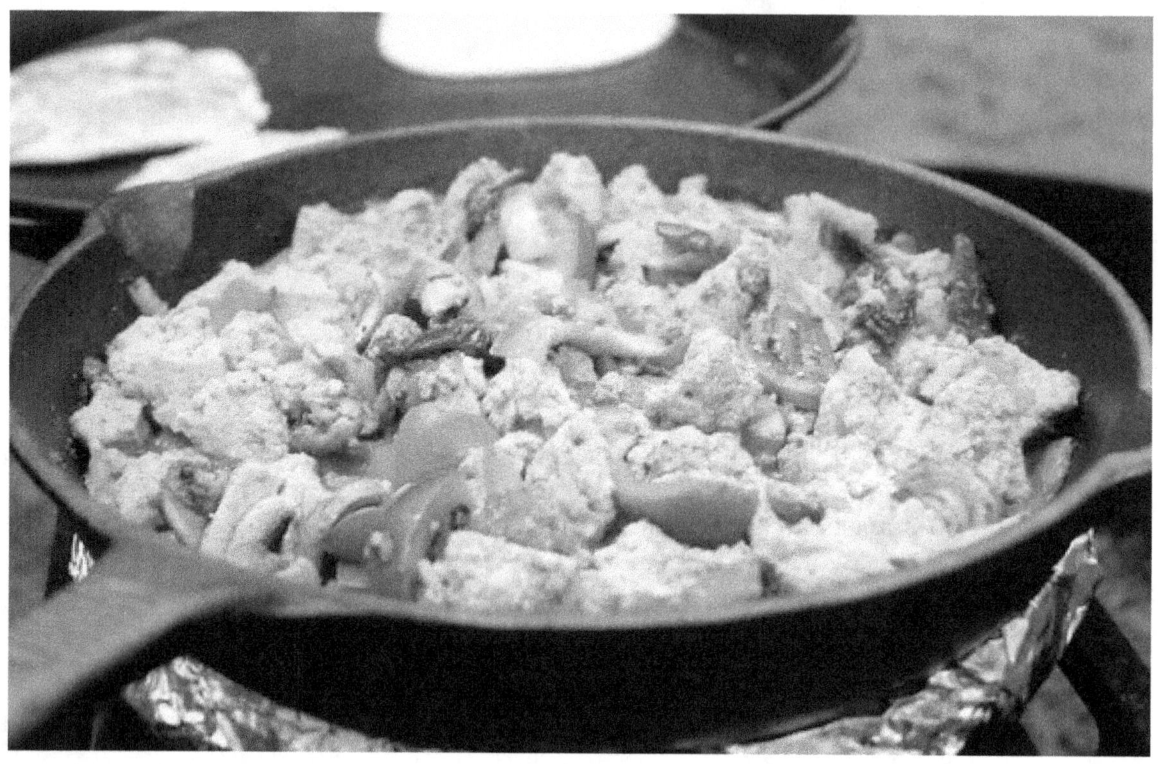

The tofu provincial is a delightful, fast, easy, and simple meal. The meal can be served along with other delicious side meals.

Servings: 2

Cooking time: 25 mins

Ingredients:

- 1 block tofu, cut into rounds
- 1 can diced tomatoes
- 4 garlic cloves
- 1 tbsp. olive oil
- 2 tsps. dried herbs
- ½ tsp. dried chili flakes
- Salt and pepper

Instructions:

1. In a skillet over a medium heat, heat the oil and cook the garlic for one minute.

2. Stir in the tomatoes, herbs, chili flakes, and salt and pepper.

3. Simmer for five minutes, then add the tofu.

4. Reduce the heat, and simmer for another fifteen minutes.

Cheese and Pesto Zoodles

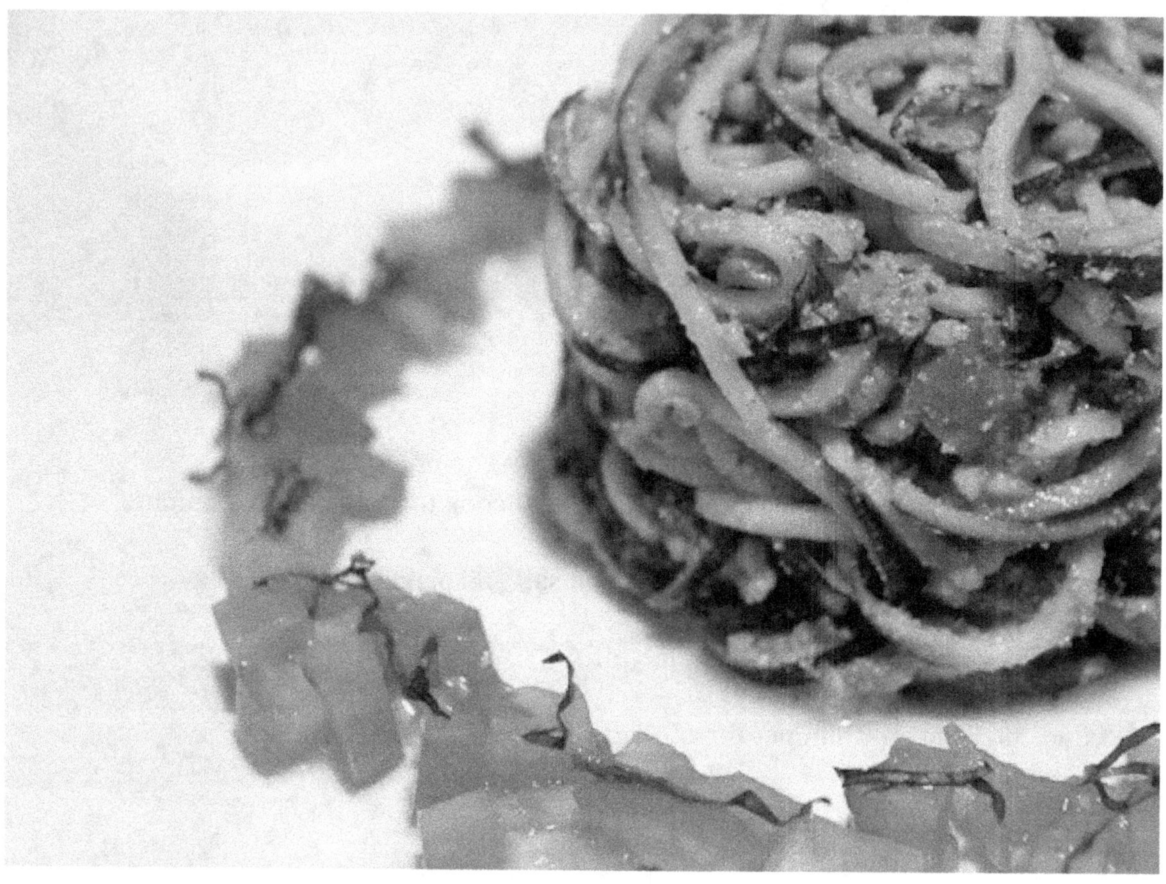

Cheese and pesto zoodles is definitely a wonderful meal that will be cherished by your family. Enjoy it.

Servings: 2

Cooking time: 20 mins

Ingredients:

- 4 c. raw zucchini noodles
- ½ c. mozzarella cheese, grated
- 1/8 c. Romano cheese, grated
- 4 oz. mascarpone cheese
- 1/8 c. parmesan cheese, grated
- 1/8 c. basil pesto
- 2 pinches nutmeg, ground
- Salt and pepper

Instructions:

1. Set your oven to 400°F and grease a casserole dish.

2. Pop the zucchini noodles into the microwave and cook on high for three minutes.

3. In a microwave safe bowl, mix the parmesan, mascarpone, and Romano cheeses with the nutmeg, and salt and pepper.

4. Microwave for one minute on high, then whisk until smooth.

5. Fold in the mozzarella cheese, basil pesto, and cooked zoodles, then pour the lot into the prepped casserole dish.

6. Cook for ten minutes, then serve immediately.

Moroccan Green Beans

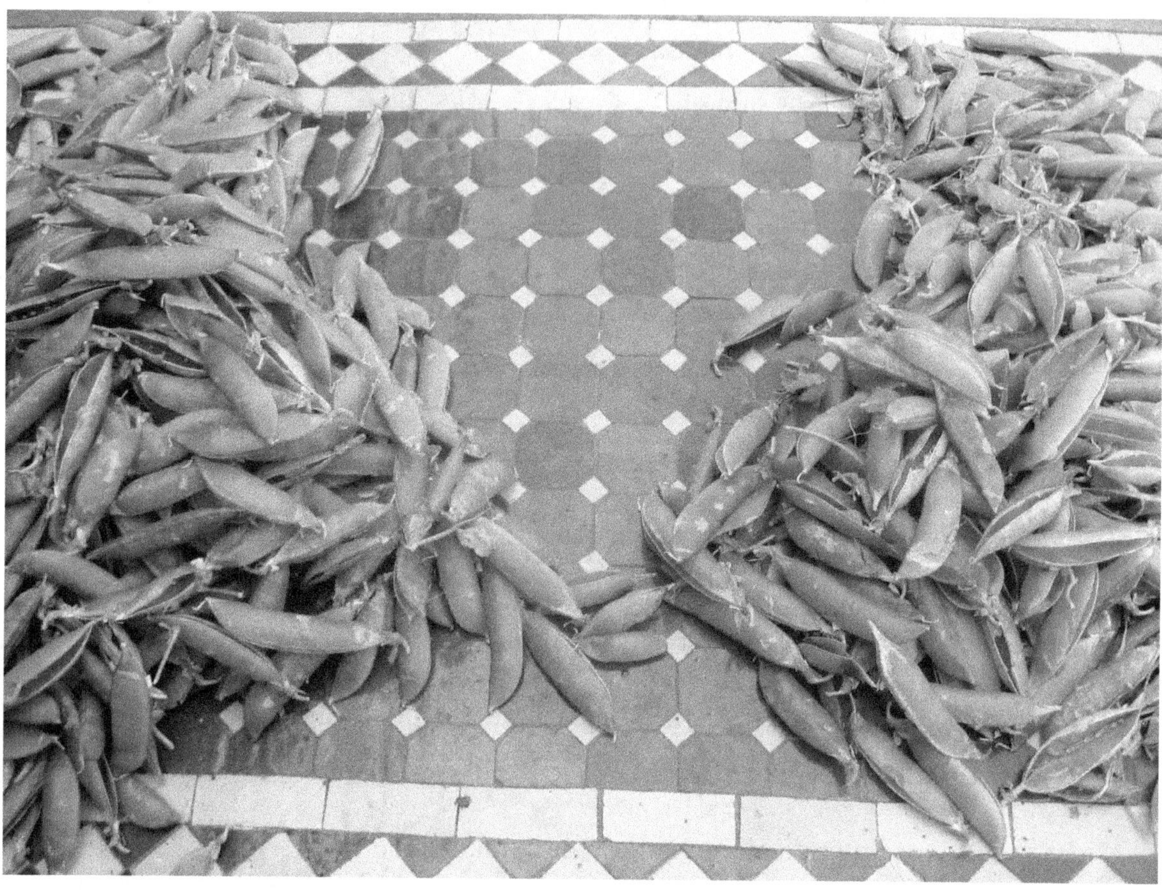

The recipe is delicious and sweet, especially when prepared in the desired way. All you need is to follow the simple preparation steps and enjoy it.

Servings: 2

Cooking time: 45 mins

Ingredients:

- 2 c. raw green beans, trimmed
- 1/3 tbsp. seasonings
- 2 tbsps. olive oil
- Salt and pepper

Instructions:

1. Take your roasting pan and apply a grease layer. Set oven to preheat at 400°F.

2. Coat the green beans in the other ingredients, then cook for twenty minutes.

3. Stir well, then cook for another ten minutes.

4. Serve warm.

Halloumi 'Bruschetta' and Tomato

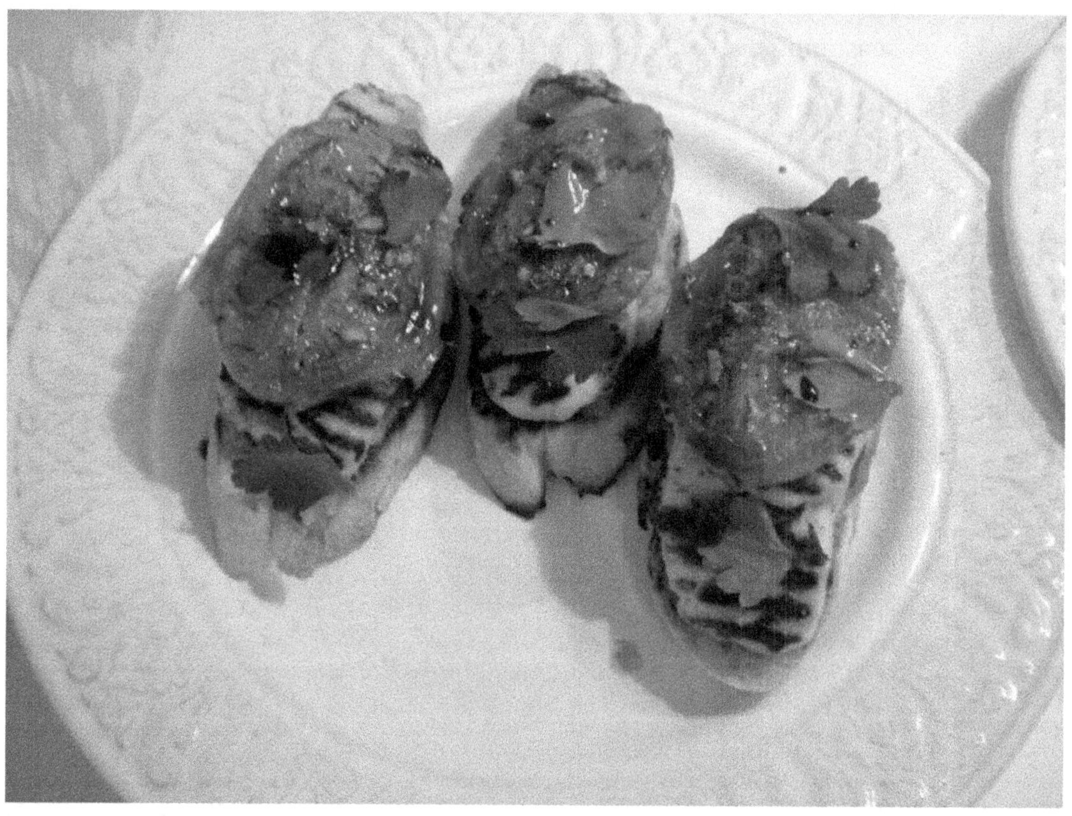

The simple Halloumi bruschetta is perfect, especially when prepared with tomato. Enjoy the flavors that come with it when topped with other desired meals.

Servings: 2

Cooking time: 20 mins

Ingredients:

- 1½ oz. sliced Halloumi cheese
- 1/3 chopped tomatoes
- ½ minced clove garlic
- 2 tbsps. Freshly chopped basil
- ½ tbsp. olive oil
- Salt and pepper

Instructions:

1. In a bowl, coat the tomatoes in the garlic, basil, olive oil, and salt and pepper.

2. Refrigerate for an hour.

3. Grill the Halloumi for two minutes per side, then top with the tomato and basil mixture.

4. Serve chilled.

Ranch Roasted Broccoli with Cheese

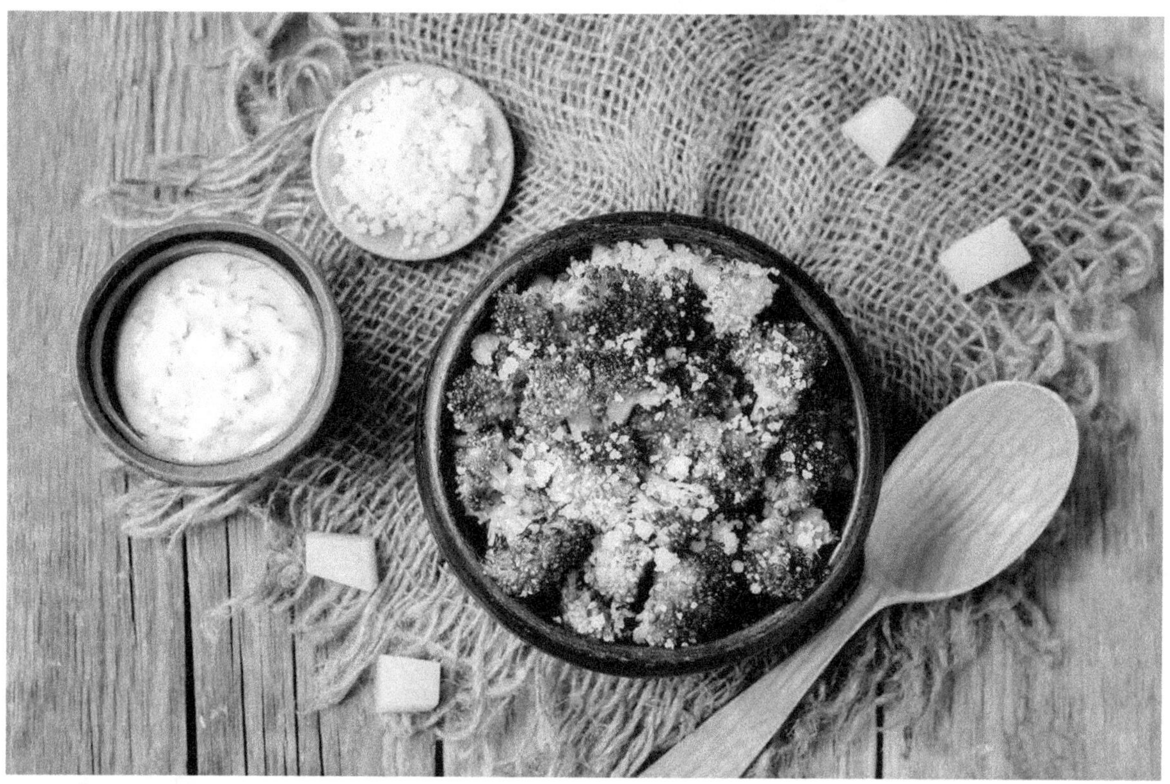

The meal is simple and easy. Enjoy it.

Servings: 2

Cooking time: 45 mins

Ingredients:

- 1½ c. broccoli florets
- 1/8 c. heavy whipping cream
- 1/8 c. ranch dressing
- ¼ c. sharp cheddar cheese, shredded
- Salt and pepper

Instructions:

1. Set your oven to preheat at 375° and grease an oven-proof casserole dish.

2. Mix everything together well, then cook in the oven for thirty minutes.

3. Serve hot.

Cauliflower Fried Rice

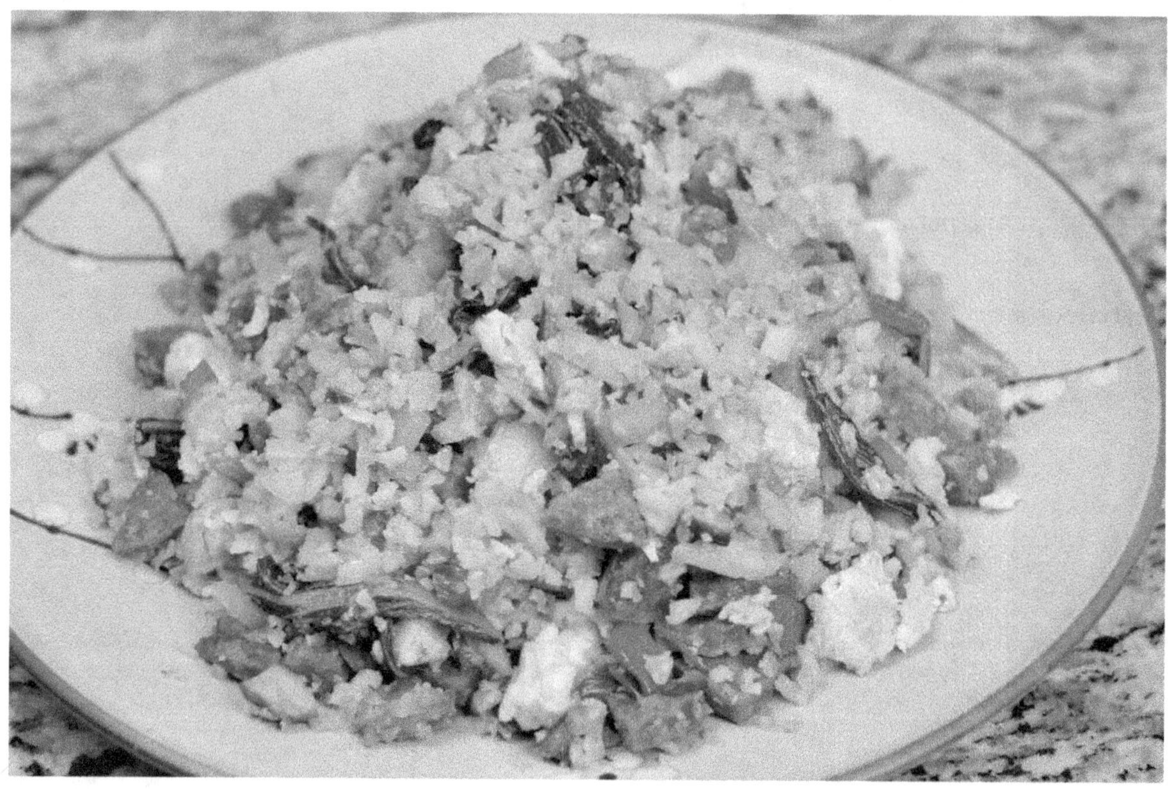

This kid friendly meal will be loved by most of your family members. Prepare it and enjoy!

Servings: 2

Cooking time: 15 mins

Ingredients:

- 6 oz. riced cauliflower, fresh or frozen
- 1 sliced green onion
- 1/8 c. diced carrots
- 1 crushed clove garlic
- 1tbsp. butter
- 1 beaten egg
- 1tbsp. soy sauce
- ½ tsp. toasted sesame oil

Instructions:

1. Adjust your heat to medium-high and set a skillet in place, melt the butter then stir in the carrots and riced cauliflower.

2. Cook for five minutes, then add the garlic and white part of the green onions and cook for another three minutes.

3. Stir in the beaten egg and cook for another two minutes.

4. Finally, stir in the soy sauce, green part of green onions, and the sesame oil.

5. Serve hot.

Whole Chicken

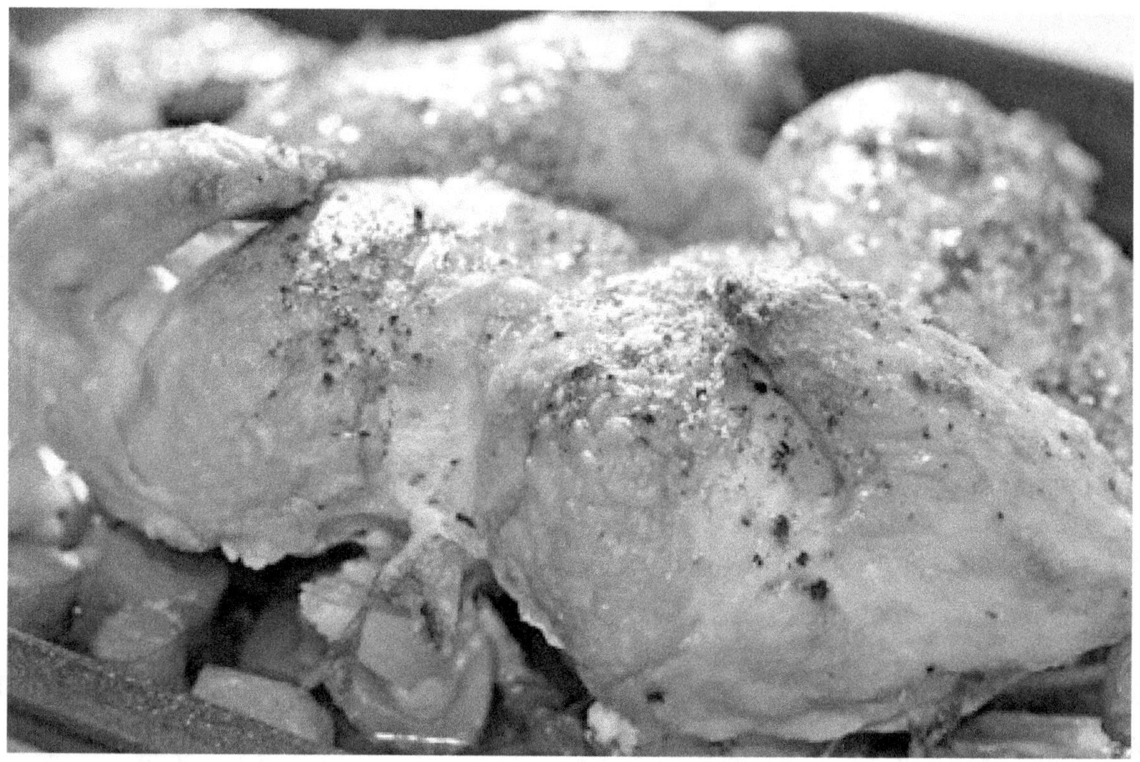

The preparation of whole chicken is much easier. You are assured of enjoying the flavor that comes with it.

Cooking time: 25 minutes

Servings: 7

Ingredients:

- 5 lbs. whole chicken
- 1 ½ tsps. Minced garlic
- 1 tbsp. Avocado oil
- 1/8 tsp. Sea salt
- ¼ tsp. Ground black pepper
- 1 sliced Lemon
- 2 c. Water
- 1 tbsp. Apple cider vinegar

Instructions:

1. Brush chicken with oil, then rub with pepper and salt and stuff its cavity with lemon slices.

2. Switch on the instant pot, pour in water, add vinegar, then place the chicken on it and shut the instant pot with its lid in the sealed position.

3. Press the 'manual' button, press '+/-' to set the cooking time to 25 minutes and cook at high-pressure setting; when the pressure builds in the pot, the cooking timer will start.

4. When the instant pot buzzes, press the 'keep warm' button, release pressure naturally for 10 minutes, then do a quick pressure release and open the lid.

5. With your cutting board ready, set on the chicken. Allow to cool before slicing. Serve.

Lamb Shanks

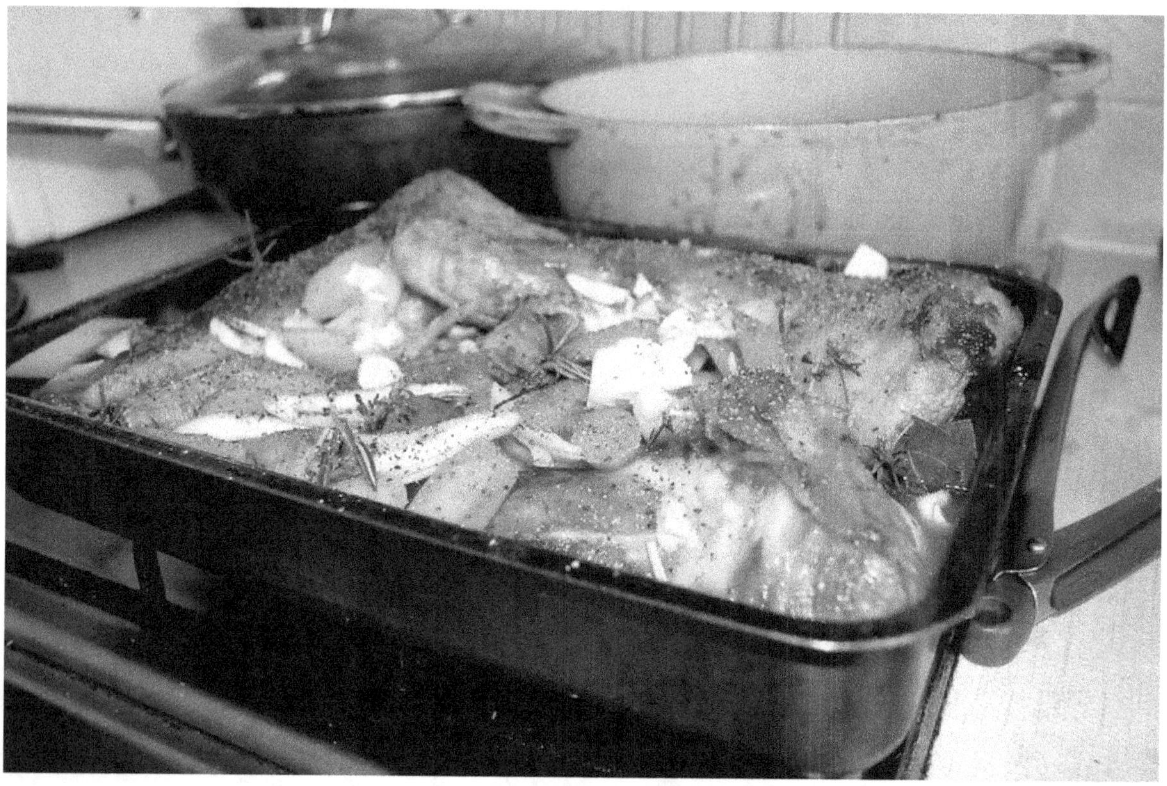

Lamb shanks are a good value to your health. A taste of them will keep you yearning for them every day.

Cooking time: 1 hour and 30 minutes

Servings: 2

Ingredients:

- ¼ c. Avocado oil
- 2.5 lbs. Lamb shanks
- 1 tbsp. Minced garlic
- 1 peeled white onion, diced
- 2 Sticks diced celery
- 2 tbsps. Rosemary
- 1 tsp. Salt
- ½ tsp. Ground black pepper
- 1 c. Lamb or chicken broth
- 14 oz. Diced tomatoes

Instructions:

1. Switch on the instant pot, add half of the oil, press the 'sauté/simmer' button, wait until the oil is hot and lamb shanks in a single layer and cook for 3 to 5 minutes per side or until browned.

2. Transfer lamb shanks to a plate, set aside, then add onion, celery, garlic, and rosemary into the instant pot and cook for 3 minutes.

3. Season with salt and black pepper, pour in the broth, mix well, then add tomatoes, return lamb shanks into the pot and toss until combined.

4. Press the 'keep warm' button, shut the instant pot with its lid in the sealed position, then press the 'manual' button, press '+/-' to set the cooking time to 50 minutes and cook at high-pressure setting; when the pressure builds in the pot, the cooking timer will start.

5. When the instant pot buzzes, press the 'keep warm' button, release pressure naturally for 10 minutes, then do a quick pressure release and open the lid.

6. Transfer lamb shanks to a dish, then press the 'sauté/simmer' button and simmer the sauce for 5 minutes or more until the sauce is reduced by half.

7. Ladle sauce over the lamb shanks and serve.

Coconut Shrimp

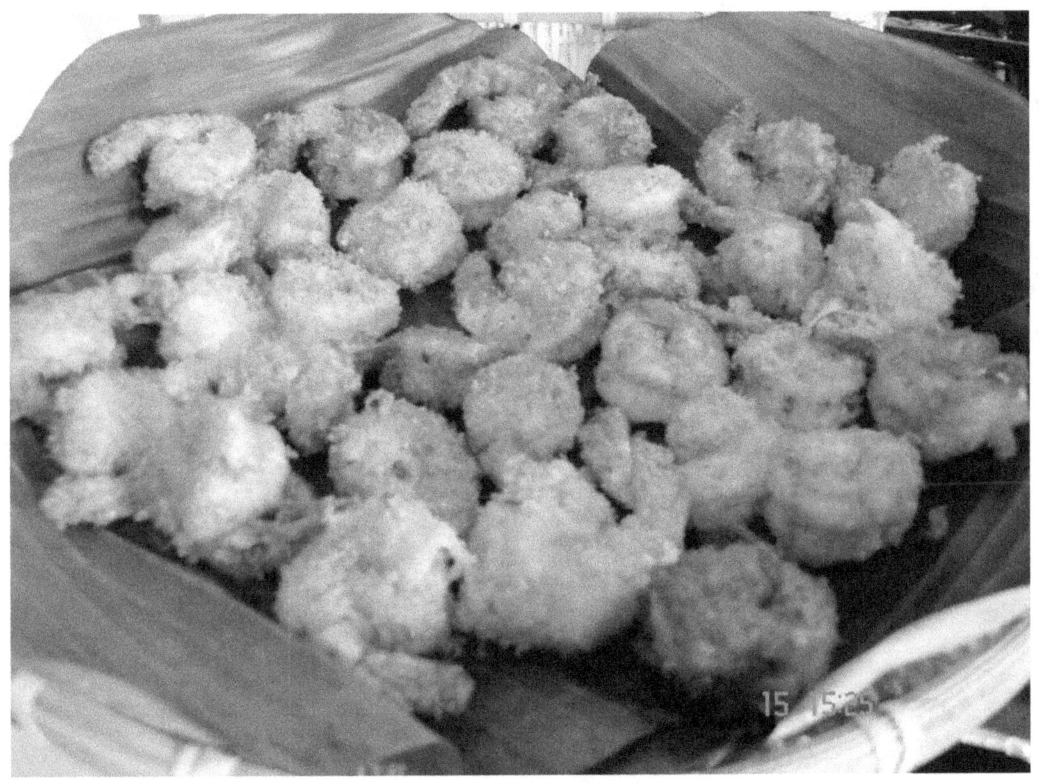

Enjoy the sweetness that comes with this coconut shrimp.

Cooking time: 12 minutes

Servings: 4

Ingredients:

- 1 lb. wild-caught deveined shrimp, peeled
- 3 tbsps. Coconut flour
- ¼ tsp. Garlic powder
- 3 beaten Eggs, Pastured
- 1 ¾ c. unsweetened Coconut flakes
- 1/8 tsp. Ground black pepper
- ¼ tsp. Smoked paprika
- ¼ tsp. Sea salt

Instructions:

1. Adjust the oven to preheat at 400 degrees F.

2. Meanwhile, crack eggs in a bowl and whisk until beaten, place coconut flakes in another dish, then place coconut flour in another dish, add salt, black pepper, garlic powder, and paprika and stir until mixed.

3. Working on one piece at a time, dredge a shrimp into the coconut flour mix, then dip into egg, and dredge with coconut flake until evenly coated.

4. Take a non-stick wire rack, line it with a baking sheet, then spray with oil and place coated shrimps on it in a single layer.

5. Place the wire rack containing shrimps into the oven, bake for 4 minutes, then flip the shrimps and continue baking for 5 to 6 minutes or until thoroughly cooked and firm.

6. Then switch on the broiler and bake the shrimps for 2 minutes or until lightly golden.

7. When done, let shrimps cooled, place them on a baking sheet in a single layer, then cover the shrimps with parchment sheet, layer with remaining shrimps and freeze until hard.

8. Then transfer shrimps into a freezer bag and store in the freezer for up to 3 months.

9. When ready to serve, reheat the shrimps at 350 degrees F for 2 to 3 minutes until hot.

Sausage Stuffed Zucchini Boats

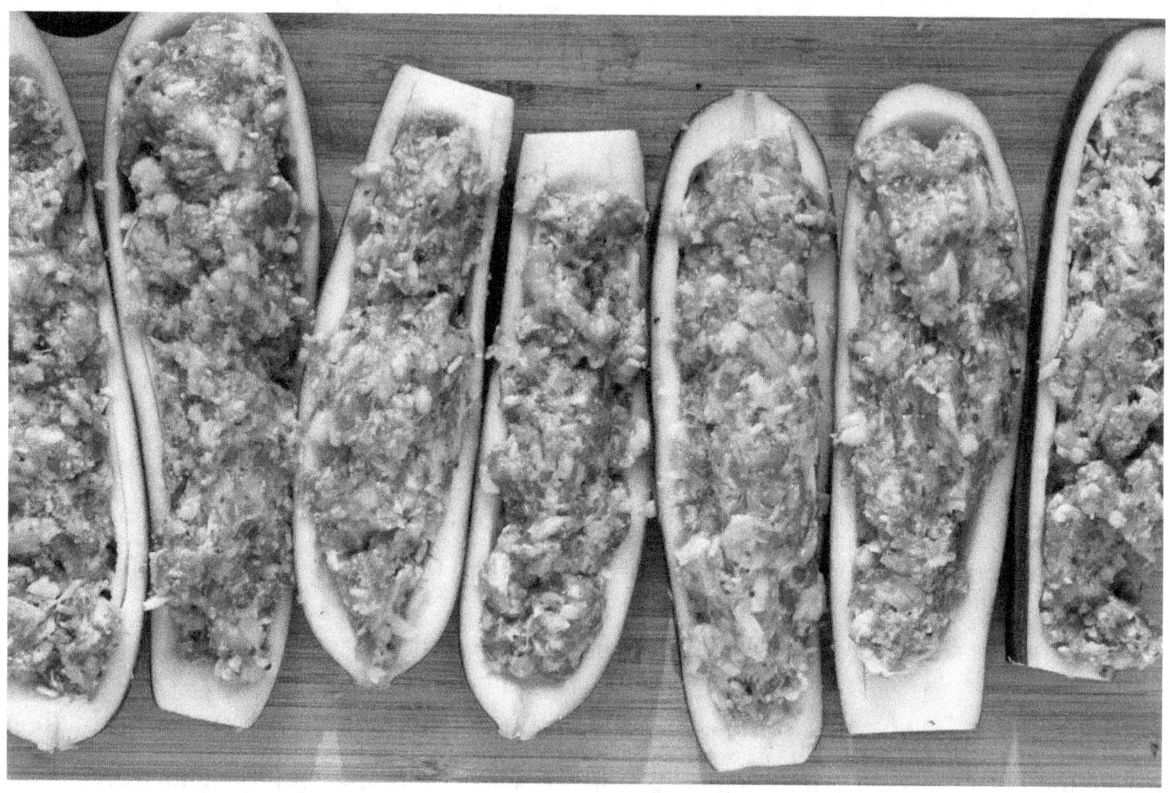

Sausage will seem much better when stuffed with zucchini boats in them. Enjoy this meal!

Cooking time: 30 minutes

Servings: 4

Ingredients:

- 4 zucchinis
- 1 lb. Ground Italian pork sausage, pastured
- 1 ½ tsp. Sea salt
- 1/3 c. peeled white onion, diced
- 1 tbsp. garlic
- 1 tsp. Italian seasoning
- 14.5 oz. Diced tomatoes
- 1/3 c. full-fat parmesan cheese, Grated
- 2 tbsps. Divided Avocado oil
- 1 c. full-fat Mozzarella cheese

Instructions:

1. Set oven to 400 degrees F and let preheat.

2. Meanwhile, cut each zucchini in half, lengthwise, then make well in the center by scooping out the centers by using a spoon.

3. Take a baking sheet, line it with parchment sheet, place zucchini halves on it, cut side up, drizzle with 1 tablespoon oil and season with salt.

4. Set into your oven and bake for 15 to 20 minutes or until soft.

5. Meanwhile, take a large skillet pan, place it over medium-high heat, add remaining oil and when hot, add onions and cook for 10 minutes until nicely brown.

6. Add sausage, stir well and cook for 5 minutes or until brown.

7. Then move sausage to one side of the pan, add garlic to the other side, cook for 1 minute or until fragrant and then mix into the sausage.

8. Remove pan from the heat, season sausage with Italian seasoning, add tomatoes and parmesan cheese, stir well and taste to adjust seasoning.

9. When zucchini halves are roasted, pat dry with paper towels, then stuff with sausage mixture.

10. Top stuffed zucchini with mozzarella cheese and bake for 5 to 10 minutes or until cheese melts, and the top is nicely golden brown.

11. Let zucchini boats cool down, then wrap each zucchini boat with an aluminum foil and freeze in the freezer.

12. When ready to serve, thaw the zucchini boat and reheat at 350 degrees F for 3 to 4 minutes until hot.

Coconut Chicken

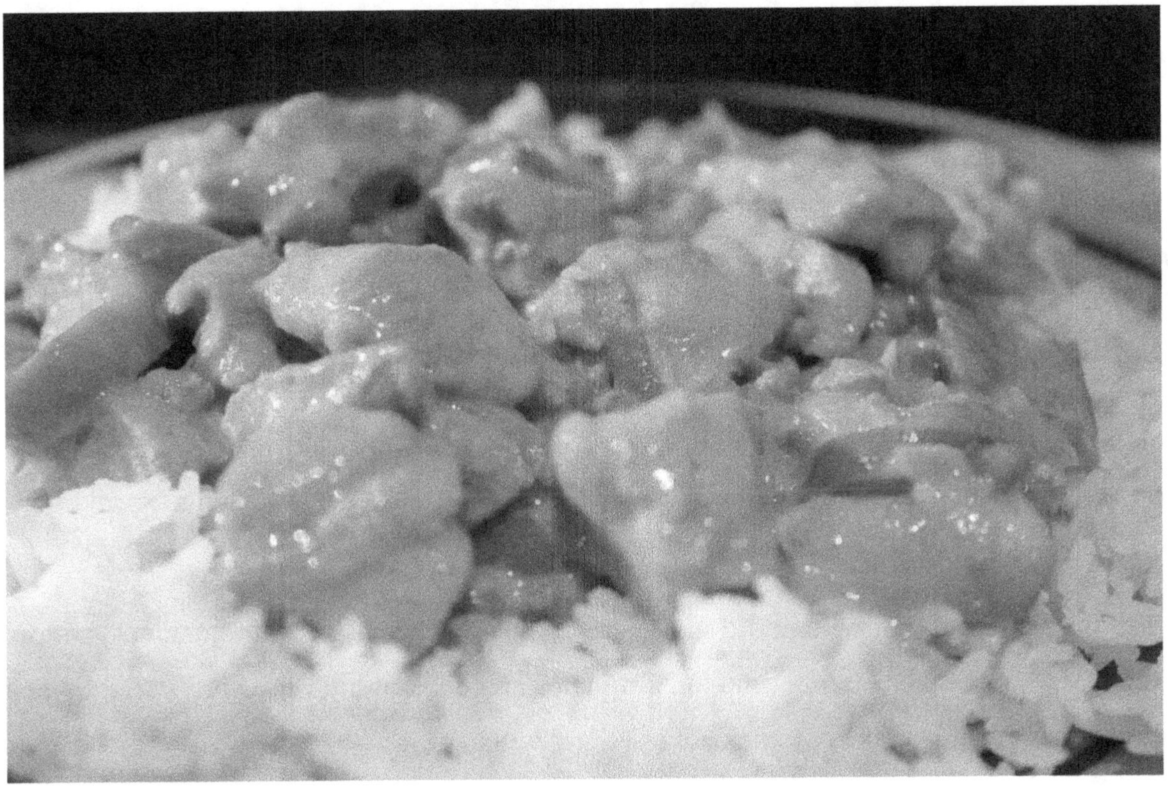

The coconut chicken will give your family a wonderful treat. Prepare it at your home and make a happy home.

Cooking time: 22 minutes

Servings: 4

Ingredients:

- 1 Bunch chopped celery
- 1 lb. cubed Chicken breast, cubed
- 1 c. Chicken broth
- 5 Stalks lemongrass
- 1 c. unsweetened Coconut milk, full-fat
- ¾ tsp. Salt
- ½ tsp. black pepper, ground

Instructions:

1. Switch on the instant pot, add celery, then top with chicken, add lemongrass and pour in chicken broth.

2. Shut the instant pot with its lid in the sealed position, then press the 'manual' button, press '+/-' to set the cooking time to 22 minutes and cook at high-pressure setting; when the pressure builds in the pot, the cooking timer will start.

3. When the instant pot buzzes, press the 'keep warm' button, do a quick pressure release and open the lid.

4. Remove and discard lemongrass, season with salt and black pepper, then pour in coconut milk and stir until combined.

5. Serve coconut chicken with cauliflower rice.

Garlic Chicken

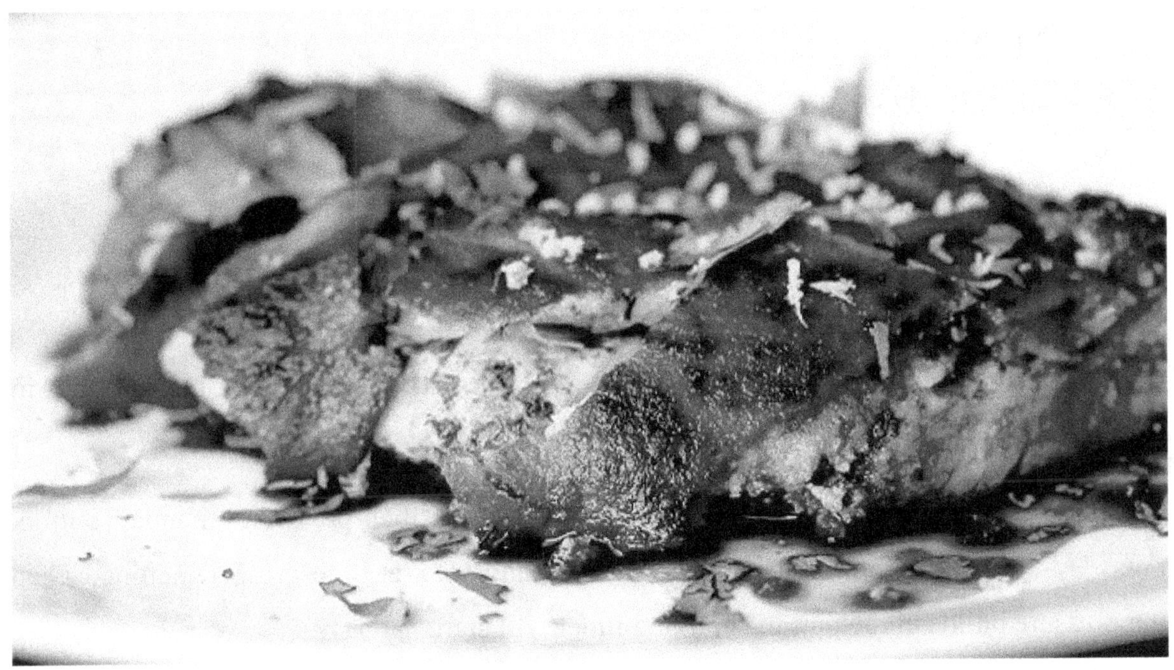

The easy and sticky garlic chicken will provide your family with all the desires of suitable food.

Cooking time: 35 minutes

Servings: 4

Ingredients:

- 4 Chicken breasts
- 1 tsp. Salt
- ¼ c. Avocado oil
- 1 tsp. Turmeric powder
- 10 Cloves garlic, peeled and diced

Instructions:

1. Switch on the instant pot, add chicken, then season with salt and black pepper, pour in the oil and scatter garlic on top.

2. Shut the instant pot with its lid in the sealed position, then press the 'manual' button, press '+/-' to set the cooking time to 35 minutes and cook at high-pressure setting; when the pressure builds in the pot, the cooking timer will start.

3. When the instant pot buzzes, press the 'keep warm' button, release pressure naturally for 10 minutes, then do a quick pressure release and open the lid.

4. Shred chicken with two forks, toss until mixed and serve as a lettuce wrap.

Desserts

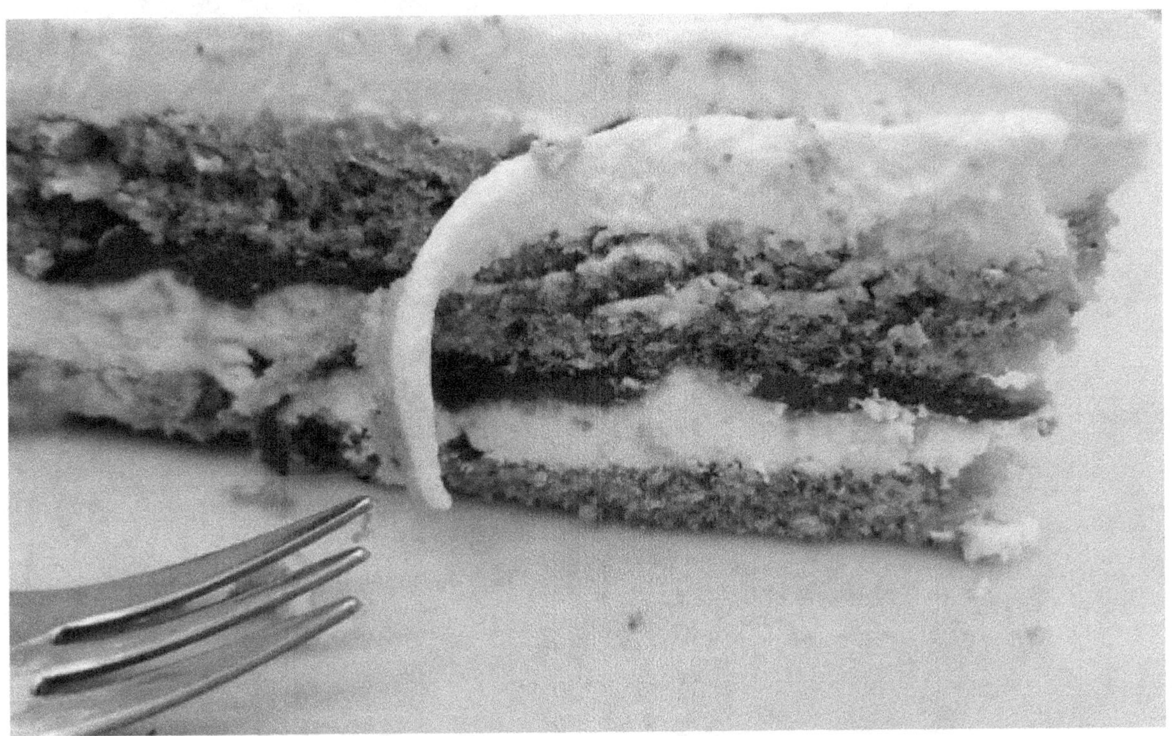

These desserts are not just like any other. The meals have special instructions that are keenly observed to maintain a diet that will be quite important for all your health needs. Enjoy them!

Thai Coconut Custard

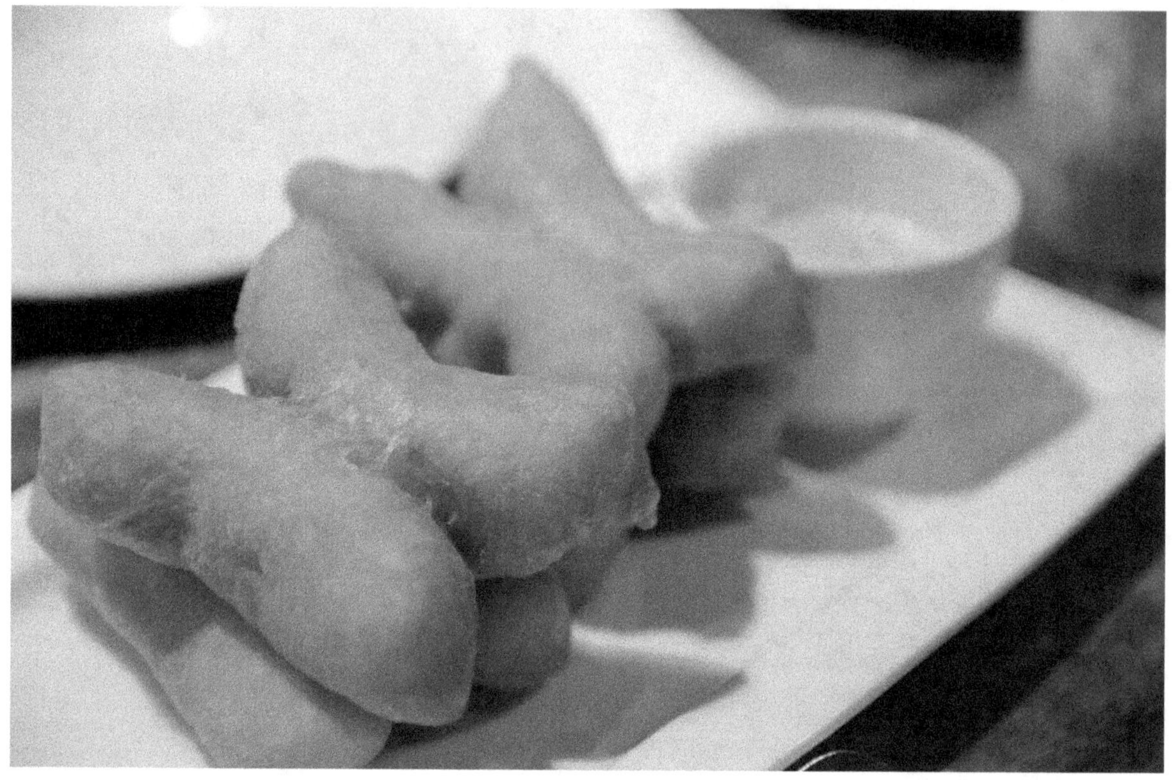

Enjoy the custard along with friends and family. It is made of ingredients that are essential to your health.

Cooking time: 30 minutes

Servings: 4

Ingredients:

- 1 c. full-fat Coconut milk
- 3 Eggs
- 1/3 c. Erythritol sweetener
- 4 drops unsweetened Vanilla extract
- 2 c. Water

Instructions:

1. Using a bowl, add in all the ingredients except for water. Blend until smooth, then pour the mixture into a 6-inch heatproof bowl and cover it with aluminum foil.

2. Switch on the instant pot, pour in water, insert trivet stand and place covered bowl on it.

3. Shut the instant pot with its lid the in the sealed position, then press the 'manual' button, press '+/-' to set the cooking time to 30 minutes and cook at high-pressure setting; when the pressure builds in the pot, the cooking timer will start.

4. When the instant pot buzzes, press the 'keep warm' button, release pressure naturally for 10 minutes, then do a quick pressure release and open the lid.

5. Take out the bowl, uncover it, and check if the custard is cooked which can be done by inserting a knife in the custard that should slide out clean.

6. Transfer the custard bowl in the refrigerator and then cool for 4 hours before serving.

Chocolate Mousse

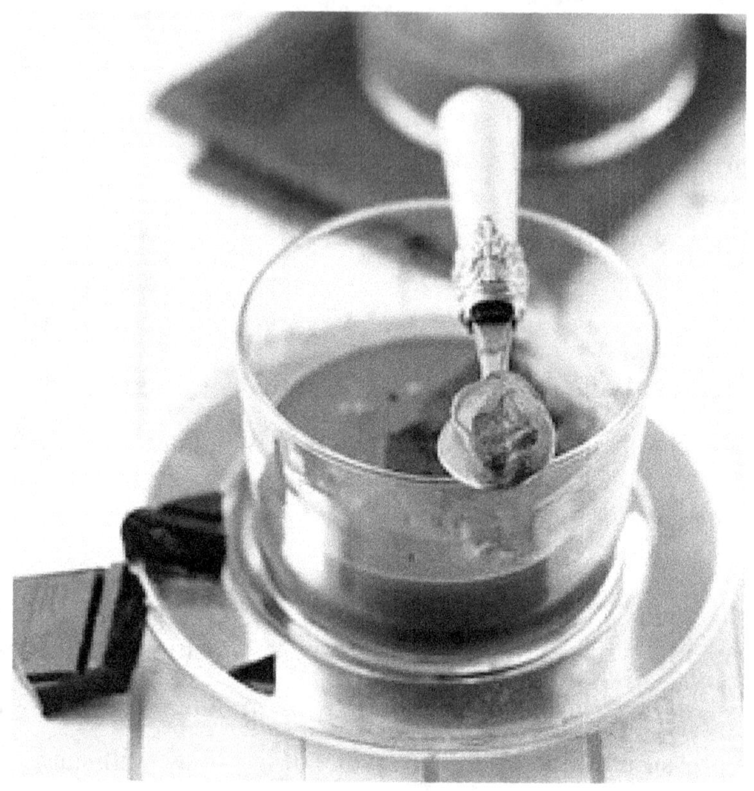

Enjoy this sweet mousse with friends and family!

Cooking time: 6 minutes

Servings: 5

Ingredients:

- 4 Egg yolks
- ½ c. Swerve sweetener
- 1 ¾ c. divided Water
- ¼ c. unsweetened Cacao powder
- 1 c. Whipping cream
- ½ c. full-fat Almond milk
- ½ tsp. unsweetened Vanilla extract
- ¼ tsp. Sea salt

Instructions:

1. Take a saucepan, add cacao and sweetener, pour in ¼ cup water, whisk until sugar is dissolved and then whisk in cream and milk until mixed.

2. Adjust your heat to medium and set the saucepan in place. Bring the mixture to a slight boil, then remove the pan from the heat, add salt and vanilla into the milk mixture and whisk well.

3. Place egg yolks in a bowl, whisk until beaten, then slowly whisk in chocolate mixture until incorporated and divide the mixture evenly between five ramekins.

4. Switch on the instant pot, pour in water, then insert a trivet stand and stack ramekins on it.

5. Shut the instant pot with its lid in the sealed position, then press the 'manual' button, press '+/-' to set the cooking time to 6 minutes and cook at high-pressure setting; when the pressure builds in the pot, the cooking timer will start.

6. When the instant pot buzzes, press the 'keep warm' button, do a quick pressure release and open the lid.

7. Take out the ramekins, let cool for 10 minutes at room temperature, then transfer them into the refrigerator and chill mousse for 4 hours.

8. Serve straight away.

Coconut Almond Cake

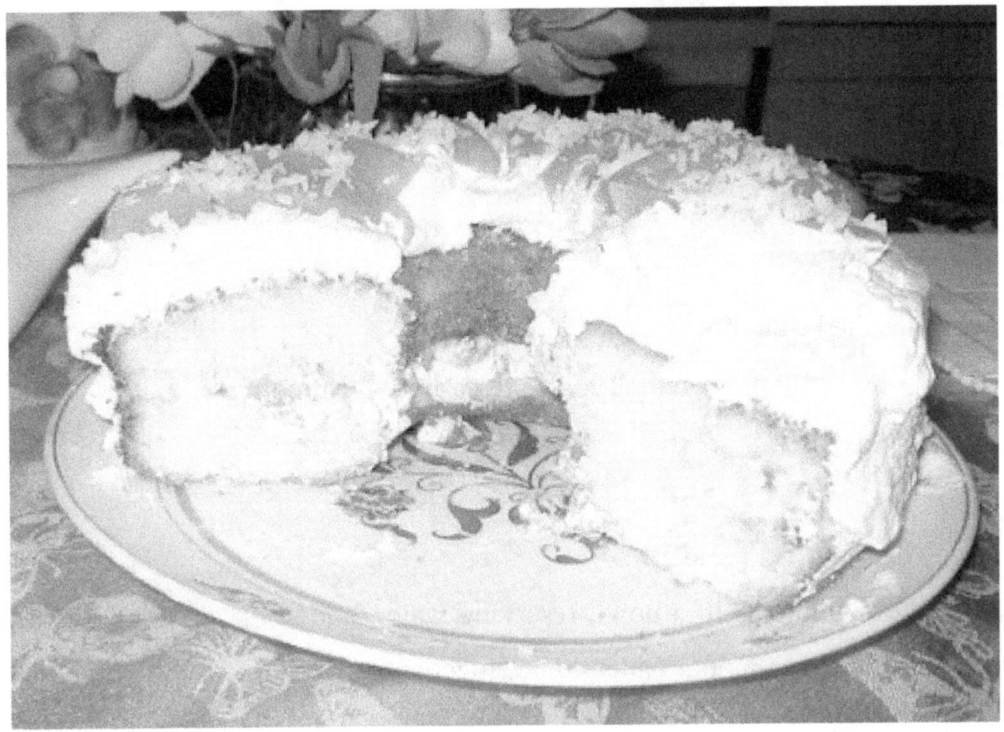

The cake is specially prepared for enjoyment of your family. Enjoy it.

Cooking time: 50 minutes

Servings: 8

Ingredients:

- 1 c. Almond flour
- ½ c. unsweetened Shredded coconut
- 1/3 c. Erythritol sweetener
- 1 tsp. Baking powder
- 1 tsp. Apple pie spice
- 2 whisked Eggs
- ¼ c. unsalted Butter, melted
- ½ c. Heavy whipping cream (you can get more for topping)
- 1 c. Water

Instructions:

1. Place all the ingredients in a bowl, reserving water, and stir well using a hand mixer until incorporated and a smooth batter comes together.

2. Take a 6-inch baking pan, spoon the prepared batter on it, then smooth the top, sprinkle with pecans and cover the pan with aluminum foil.

3. Switch on the instant pot, pour in water, insert a trivet stand and place pan on it.

4. Shut the instant pot with its lid in the sealed position, then press the 'cake' button, press '+/-' to set the cooking time to 40 minutes and cook at high-pressure setting; when the pressure builds in the pot, the cooking timer will start.

5. When the instant pot buzzes, press the 'keep warm' button, release pressure naturally for 10 minutes, then do a quick pressure release and open the lid.

6. Take out the pan, uncover it, invert the pan on a plate to take out the cake and let cool for 15 minutes.

7. Spread cream on top of the cake, then cut into slices and serve.

Chocolate Muffins

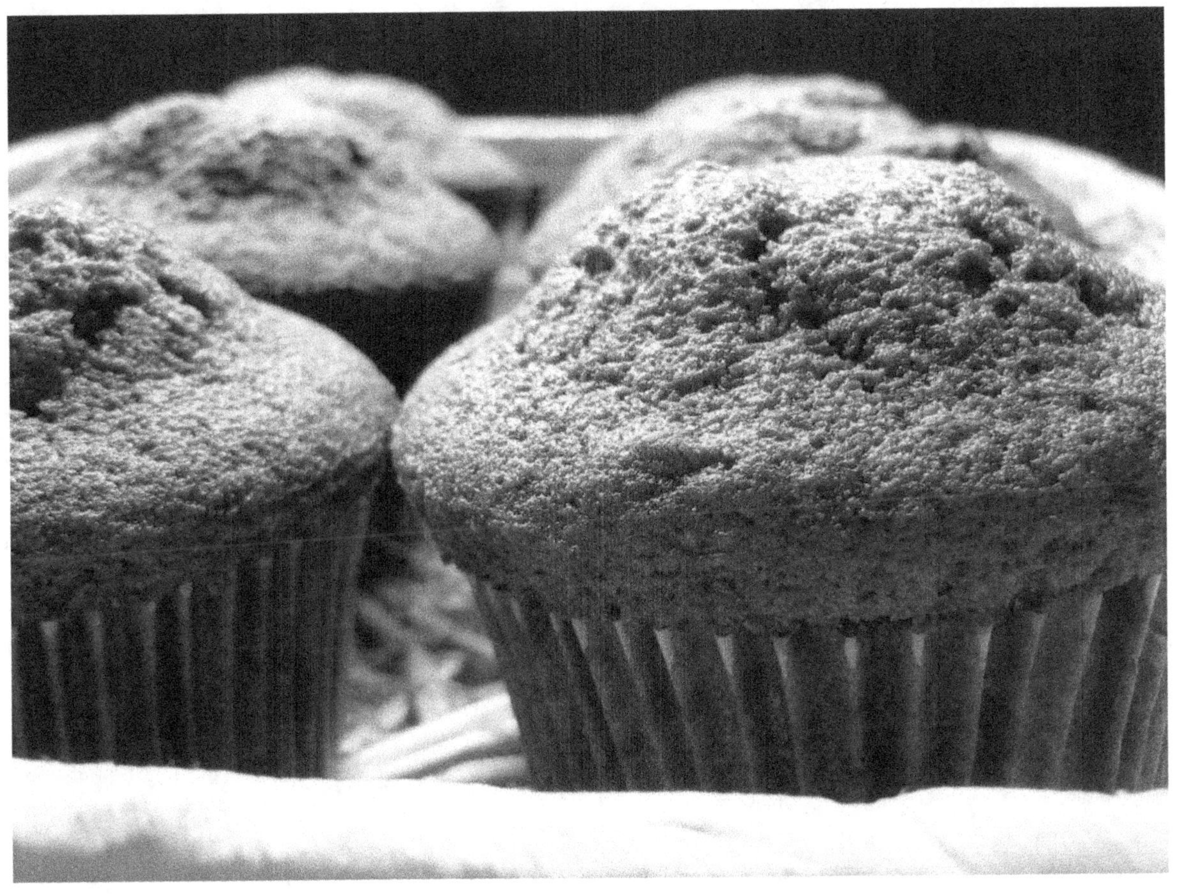

Try out the chocolate. You are definitely ensured of having the flavor of a Keto meal of your desire.

Cooking time: 45 minutes

Servings: 8 muffins

Ingredients:

- 2 c. chopped Pumpkin, steamed
- ½ c. Coconut flour
- 1/8 tsp. Salt
- 4 tbsps. Erythritol sweetener
- 1 c. Cacao powder, unsweetened
- ½ c. Collagen protein powder
- 1 tsp. Baking soda
- 4.6 oz. melted Cacao butter
- ½ c. Avocado oil
- 2 tsps. Apple cider vinegar
- 3 tsps. Unsweetened Vanilla extract
- 3 pastured Eggs

Instructions:

1. Set oven to 350 degrees F and let preheat until muffins are ready to bake.

2. Add all the ingredients in a food processor or blender, except for collagen, and pulse for 1 to 2 minutes or until well combined and incorporated.

3. Then add collagen and pulse at low speed until just mixed.

4. Take an eight cups silicon muffin tray, grease the cups with avocado oil and then evenly scoop the prepared batter in them.

5. Place the muffin tray into the oven and bake the muffins for 30 minutes or until thoroughly cooked and a knife inserted into each muffin comes out clean.

6. When done, let muffins cool in the pan for 10 minutes, then take them out from the tray and cool on the wire rack.

7. Place muffins in the large freezer bag or wrap each muffin with a foil and store them in the refrigerator for four days or in freezer for up to 3 months.

8. When ready to serve, microwave muffins for 45 seconds to 1 minute or until thoroughly heated and then serve with coconut cream.

Conclusion

You have a powerful weight-loss tool in your hands. Be sure to read and follow the entire recommended instructions in this manual. As evident from this manual, you can have your favorite and delicious meals even while on the Keto diet. As long as it is not processed foods and the carb content is reasonable, you have no problem. Remove restriction from your mind and tap into your creativity to come up with amazing meals you can enjoy on a diet.

Let your goal be your driving force. Try out all the recipes. Good luck!

About the Author

Angel Burns learned to cook when she worked in the local seafood restaurant near her home in Hyannis Port in Massachusetts as a teenager. The head chef took Angel under his wing and taught the young woman the tricks of the trade for cooking seafood. The skills she had learned at a young age helped her get accepted into Boston University's Culinary Program where she also minored in business administration.

Summers off from school meant working at the same restaurant but when Angel's mentor and friend retired as head chef, she took over after graduation and created classic and new dishes that delighted the diners. The restaurant flourished under Angel's culinary creativity and one customer developed more than an appreciation for Angel's food. Several months after taking over the position, the young woman met her future husband at work and they have been inseparable ever since. They still live in Hyannis Port with their two children and a cocker spaniel named Buddy.

Angel Burns turned her passion for cooking and her business acumen into a thriving e-book business. She has authored several successful books on cooking different types of dishes using simple ingredients for novices and experienced chefs alike. She is still head chef in Hyannis Port and says she will probably never leave!

Author's Afterthoughts

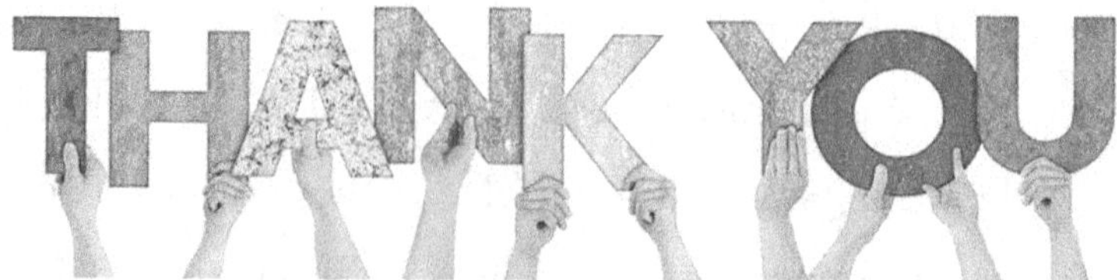

With so many books out there to choose from, I want to thank you for choosing this one and taking precious time out of your life to buy and read my work. Readers like you are the reason I take such passion in creating these books.

It is with gratitude and humility that I express how honored I am to become a part of your life and I hope that you take the same pleasure in reading this book as I did in writing it.

Can I ask one small favour? I ask that you write an honest and open review on Amazon of what you thought of the book. This will help other readers make an informed choice on whether to buy this book.

My sincerest thanks,

Angel Burns

If you want to be the first to know about news, new books, events and giveaways, subscribe to my newsletter by clicking the link below

https://angel-burns.gr8.com

or Scan QR-code